Queer Magic: Spells for Love, Protection & Empowerment

Everyday Witchcraft for LGBTQ+ Lives

Alex Wren

This book is dedicated to all the LGBTQ+ folks who dare to live magically, authentically, and boldly. Your courage creates possibilities for generations to come.

Copyright © 2025 by Alex Wren

All rights reserved.

No part of this book may be reproduced, stored in a retrieval system, or transmitted in any form or by any means—electronic, mechanical, photocopying, recording, or otherwise—without the prior written permission of the publisher, except for brief quotations in critical reviews or articles.

ISBN 978-1-918219-11-1

First Edition: 2025

Published by: Cosmic Jive Publishing
www.cosmicjivepublishing.com

Disclaimer: The views expressed in this book are solely those of the author and do not necessarily reflect the official policy or position of the publisher.

The contents of this book are for entertainment and educational purposes only. The practices, spells, and rituals described within are based on folklore, tradition, and personal interpretation. Results may vary, and no guarantees are made regarding their efficacy. Always exercise caution, personal responsibility, and respect for others when engaging in magical practices. The author and publisher are not liable for any consequences, direct or indirect, arising from the use or misuse of this material. Magic is a personal journey—trust your intuition and act with integrity.

ABOUT THE AUTHOR

The author is a practicing magical worker and longtime member of the LGBTQ+ community who has been integrating queerness and spirituality for over a decade. Having navigated their own journey of coming out, building chosen family, and creating authentic magical practice in a world that doesn't always make space for either queerness or magic, they understand firsthand the unique challenges and extraordinary gifts that come with living at the intersection of these identities.

Their magical practice draws from multiple traditions including folk magic, modern witchcraft, and energy work, always filtered through the lens of lived LGBTQ+ experience. They have facilitated workshops on queer spirituality, mentored young LGBTQ+ folks exploring magical practice, and been active in creating inclusive spiritual communities both online and in their local area.

As someone who has experienced the transformative power of magic in navigating everything from workplace discrimination to family acceptance to gender expression, they are passionate about making magical practice accessible to LGBTQ+ folks at all stages of their journey. They believe deeply that queerness and magic are natural allies – both require courage to live authentically, both involve transformation and self-determination, and both offer powerful tools for creating positive change in the world.

When not writing about magic or facilitating community gatherings, they can be found tending their herb garden, reading tarot for friends, volunteering with local LGBTQ+ organizations, or experimenting with new spell recipes in their kitchen. They live with their chosen family (both human and feline) and believe that the most powerful magic happens when people are free to be completely themselves.

This book represents years of magical practice, community building, and the deep conviction that every LGBTQ+ person deserves access to spiritual tools that honor their authentic identity and support their highest good. They hope it serves as both practical guide and loving reminder that your queerness is not something to overcome in your spiritual practice – it's one of your greatest magical strengths.

"Magic taught me that transformation is not only possible but sacred. My queerness taught me that authenticity is revolutionary. Together, they've shown me that living as your true self is the most powerful spell you can cast."

Contents

Introduction — 7

Chapter 1
Magic Is Already Queer (And You Already Are Too) — 11

Chapter 2
Protection Magic for Queer Lives — 20

Chapter 3
Love Magic That Actually Works — 33

Chapter 4
Career and Money Magic — 48

Chapter 5
Gender Magic and Body Blessings — 62

Chapter 6
Community and Celebration Magic — 78

Chapter 7
Everyday Magic for Extraordinary Lives — 94

Chapter 8
Building Your Long-Term Practice — 110

Appendix and Final Thoughts — 126

INTRODUCTION
Welcome to Your Magical Journey

Hey beautiful human,

If you've picked up this book, chances are you're looking for something the mainstream magical world hasn't quite offered you yet. Maybe you've wandered through crystal shops where everything feels very... straight and narrow. Perhaps you've read spell books that assume everyone wants the same things from love magic, or that everyone's relationship with their body and gender is simple and settled.

Well, welcome to a different kind of magic book.

This is magic for people who know that identity can be fluid, that families can be chosen, that love comes in countless beautiful forms, and that sometimes the most magical thing you can do is simply show up authentically in a world that would prefer you didn't. This is magic that honors all the parts of you – the parts you celebrate, the parts you're still figuring out, and the parts that change as you grow.

I'm not going to assume anything about your spiritual background, your relationship status, your pronouns, or your living situation. What I will assume is that you're here because you want to tap into something powerful within yourself, and you want magical practices that actually fit your real, gloriously complicated, authentically queer life.

What This Book Is (And Isn't)

This book is a practical guide to magic that works with your lived experience as an LGBTQ+ person. It's full of spells you can do with things you probably already have, rituals that fit into busy schedules, and magical thinking that makes sense when your life doesn't fit neat categories.

This isn't a book about the history of witchcraft (though we'll touch on how magical traditions have always included queer folks). It's not going to require you to spend hundreds of dollars on supplies or dedicate hours to elaborate rituals. And it's definitely not going to tell you there's only one right way to be magical.

What it will do is give you tools that work. Real, practical magic for real, practical problems.

A Note on Safety

Before we dive in, let's talk about something important: your safety matters more than any spell ever could. Magic is amazing, but it's not a replacement for practical precautions, medical care, or legal protections. If you're in an unsafe situation – whether that's an abusive relationship, a hostile workplace, or a family that won't accept you – please reach out for concrete help alongside any magical work you do.

That said, magic can be an incredible tool for building confidence, processing emotions, manifesting positive changes, and connecting with your inner strength. It's a complement to therapy, activism, and practical planning – not a replacement for them.

Your Magic, Your Rules

Throughout this book, you'll notice I give lots of suggestions but very few absolute rules. That's intentional.

The most powerful magic is the kind that feels authentic to you. If a spell calls for lavender but you can't stand the smell, use something else. If a ritual suggests dancing naked under the full moon but you live in a studio apartment with thin walls, adapt it. Your practice should fit your life, not the other way around.

The magic in these pages is meant to be a starting point. Take what resonates, leave what doesn't, and don't be afraid to modify everything to suit your needs. Trust your intuition – it's the most important magical tool you have.

CHAPTER 1
MAGIC IS ALREADY QUEER
(AND YOU ALREADY ARE TOO)

Let's start with something that might surprise you: magic has always been queer.

I don't just mean that LGBTQ+ folks have always been drawn to magical practices (though we absolutely have). I mean that magic itself – the real, transformative, life-changing stuff – operates on principles that are fundamentally queer.

Think about it: magic is about transformation, about becoming something new, about defying categories and expectations. It's about finding power in places mainstream society says there shouldn't be any. It's about creating your own rules and trusting your inner knowing over external authorities. Sound familiar?

The same forces that drive people to come out, to transition, to love boldly and authentically – those are magical forces. The courage it takes to live as your true self in a world that often punishes authenticity? That's not just brave. That's literally magical.

Reclaiming What Was Always Ours

For centuries, the people society pushed to the margins – including many of our queer ancestors – were often the ones who kept magical traditions alive. We were the wise women and cunning folk, the healers and shamans, the ones who lived between worlds and understood that reality is far more fluid than most people want to admit.

Then, as magical practices became more commercialized and mainstream, they also became sanitized. Straightened out, you might say. Magic got packaged as lifestyle content for suburban witches, with an emphasis on traditional gender roles, nuclear family structures, and very specific ideas about what "normal" relationships should look like.

But here's the thing: that was never what magic was really about. Real magic – the transformative, powerful, life-changing kind – has always been the domain of people who couldn't or wouldn't fit into neat little boxes.

So when you practice magic as a queer person, you're not appropriating something that doesn't belong to you. You're reclaiming something that was always yours.

YOUR QUEER MAGICAL ADVANTAGES

Being LGBTQ+ actually gives you some significant advantages as a magical practitioner:

You're already comfortable with transformation.

Whether you've gone through the process of coming out, transitioning, or simply evolving in your understanding of yourself, you know that identity can be fluid and that change – even scary change – can be profoundly positive.

You understand that reality is subjective.

You've probably had the experience of living in a world where most people see you one way while you know you're something entirely different. That experience of holding multiple truths simultaneously is exactly what magic requires.

You're practiced at creating your own meaning.

When the scripts society offers don't fit your life, you learn to write your own. That's essentially what magic is – creating meaning, purpose, and power outside of mainstream structures.

You know that small acts can be revolutionary.

Holding your partner's hand, using your chosen name, wearing clothes that feel right – these everyday acts can be radical. Magic works the same way. Small, intentional actions can create massive shifts.

You're comfortable with mystery.

If you've ever struggled with questions of identity, attraction, or belonging, you know that not everything can be neatly categorized or fully explained. Magic requires comfort with ambiguity and mystery.

SETTING UP YOUR PRACTICE

Now, let's talk practical matters. How do you actually start a magical practice that honors your queer identity?

First, forget everything you think you know about what magical practitioners are "supposed" to look like or do. There's no right way to be magical, just like there's no right way to be queer.

Start with intention, not stuff.

You don't need a perfect altar, expensive crystals, or rare

herbs to practice magic. You need clear intention and the willingness to pay attention to what happens when you set that intention in motion.

Make space that feels safe.

Whether that's a corner of your bedroom, a spot in your garden, or just a special notebook you keep your magical thoughts in, create space that feels authentically yours. This might look very different from the Instagram-worthy altars you see online, and that's perfect.

BASIC TOOLS AND SUPPLIES

Here's what you actually need to get started (spoiler alert: it's way less than you think):

Something to write with and write on.

A journal, notebook, or even your phone's notes app. Magic works better when you record what you do and what happens.

Candles or another source of fire.

Even a lighter counts. Fire represents transformation and energy.

Salt or another cleansing agent.

Salt is traditional, but you can use baking soda, moon water, or even visualization if physical cleansing isn't possible.

A cup or bowl.

For holding water, offerings, or spell ingredients.

Your intuition.

This is the most important tool, and you already have it.
Everything else – crystals, herbs, tarot cards, fancy ritual tools – can be added as you discover what appeals to you. But they're extras, not essentials.

CREATING SACRED SPACE

In magical terms, "sacred space" is simply space where you feel connected to something larger than yourself and free to be your most authentic self. For queer folks, this might be more about emotional safety than elaborate rituals.
Here are some simple ways to create sacred space:

Physical cleansing.

Light a candle, burn some incense, or sprinkle salt water around your space. The physical act helps signal to your brain that something special is about to happen.

Emotional boundaries.

Take a few deep breaths and set an intention to leave stress, judgment, and outside expectations outside your magical space. This is your time to connect with your authentic self.

Inviting in support.

This might be spirits, guides, ancestors, or simply your own highest self. Some people like to call on specific deities;

others prefer to work with more abstract forces like love, courage, or wisdom.

Setting intention.

Be clear about what you're hoping to accomplish. This doesn't have to be elaborate – even something like "I'm here to connect with my inner wisdom" or "I want to feel more confident in who I am" works perfectly.

The most important thing is that sacred space feels safe and authentic to you. Trust your instincts about what that looks like.

WORKING WITH ENERGY

At its core, magic is about working with energy – your own energy, the energy of objects and places, and the energy of intention and desire. As queer folks, we often have a lot of experience with energy management, even if we don't think of it in magical terms.

Think about coming out: you probably spent time building up courage (raising energy), choosing your moment carefully (timing), and then releasing that energy through the act of telling your truth. That's essentially what all magic does – it raises, focuses, and releases energy toward a specific goal.

Here are some basic energy-working techniques that will serve you well in magical practice:

Grounding.

This means connecting with stable, supportive energy – usually by visualizing roots growing from your feet into the earth, or by focusing on your breath. Grounding helps you stay centered during magical work and prevents you from feeling scattered afterward.

Shielding.

Visualizing protective energy around yourself, like a bubble of light or a cloak of safety. This is especially useful before challenging situations or when you're feeling emotionally vulnerable.

Raising energy.

This can be done through movement, chanting, drumming, or simply focusing intently on your goal. The key is to build up emotional intensity in a controlled way.

Releasing energy.

Once you've raised energy toward your magical goal, you need to release it so it can do its work. This might mean blowing out a candle, burying a spell bag, or simply stating "so mote it be" and letting go of attachment to the outcome.

ETHICS AND RESPONSIBILITY

Magic raises questions about ethics and responsibility. When is it okay to influence other people through magical means? How do you handle situations where your desires might conflict with someone else's free will?

These questions don't have simple answers, but here are some guidelines that work well for queer magical practitioners:

Focus on yourself first.

The most effective magic usually works on your own energy, confidence, and circumstances rather than trying to directly control other people.

Consider harm carefully.

The old rule "harm none" is a good starting point, but it's worth remembering that sometimes preventing greater harm requires accepting smaller harms. Use your judgment.

Respect consent.

Doing magic to help someone without their knowledge or consent is generally not a good idea, even if your intentions are loving.

Take responsibility for your impact.

Magic has consequences, just like any other action. Be prepared to own the results of your magical work.

Remember that you have agency.

You always have the right to protect yourself, pursue your happiness, and create positive change in your life. Don't let anyone convince you that it's selfish or wrong to use magic for your own benefit.

STARTING SIMPLE

Your first magical experiments should be small, low-stakes, and focused on things you genuinely care about. Here are some ideas:

Protection visualization.

When you're heading into a potentially uncomfortable situation, spend a few minutes visualizing yourself surrounded by protective light. Set the intention that you'll be safe and that any negativity directed toward you will bounce off harmlessly.

Gratitude magic.

At the end of each day, think of three things you're genuinely grateful for and imagine sending loving energy toward them. This simple practice can shift your overall energy toward positivity and abundance.

Cleansing ritual.

When you're feeling emotionally heavy or drained, take a shower or bath with the intention of washing away negativity and stress. Visualize the water carrying away anything that doesn't serve you.

These might seem almost too simple to be "real" magic, but that's exactly the point. The most powerful magic often looks deceptively ordinary from the outside. What makes it magical is the intention, attention, and energy you bring to it.

CHAPTER 2
Protection Magic for Queer Lives

Let's be honest: the world can be challenging for LGBTQ+ folks. Whether it's workplace discrimination, family rejection, street harassment, or just the constant low-level stress of wondering whether it's safe to be yourself in any given situation, we often need protection magic that goes beyond generic "shield yourself from negativity" spells.

This chapter is about practical protection magic for real situations queer people face. We'll cover everything from everyday shielding to specific protections for work, dating, and family situations.

DAILY SHIELDING: YOUR MAGICAL ARMOR

Think of daily shielding like putting on clothes – it's basic protection you probably want to have in place most of the time. The goal isn't to wall yourself off from the world, but to create a buffer that lets positive energy in while filtering out hostility, judgment, and other people's baggage.

The Rainbow Shield Visualization

This is a simple but powerful daily protection technique that honors your queer identity while providing practical protection.

What you need: Just yourself and a few minutes of quiet

time *Best time:* Morning, as part of your getting-ready routine

Sit or stand comfortably and close your eyes. Take three deep breaths, allowing your body to relax with each exhale.

Visualize a warm, golden light beginning to glow in your heart center. This light represents your authentic self – all the parts of your identity that make you who you are.

Watch as this light expands, growing brighter and stronger. As it grows, it begins to show all the colors of the rainbow – red for courage and passion, orange for creativity and joy, yellow for wisdom and confidence, green for growth and healing, blue for truth and communication, indigo for intuition and inner knowing, and violet for spiritual connection and transformation.

Let this rainbow light expand until it surrounds your entire body in a bubble of colorful, protective energy. Set the intention that this shield will:

- Allow love, respect, and positive energy to flow freely in and out
- Deflect hostility, judgment, and discrimination
- Help you recognize safe people and situations
- Remind you of your own inherent worth and power

When you're ready, open your eyes and go about your day, knowing you're protected.

The Invisible Crown

This technique is perfect for situations where you need to feel confident and protected but want to be subtle about it.

Visualize an invisible crown of light on your head. This crown represents your inherent dignity and worth as a human being. It reminds you that you belong wherever you are and that you deserve respect.

The crown can be as simple or elaborate as you like – a simple band of white light, an ornate creation with jewels and symbols that represent your identity, or anything in between. The important thing is that it feels right to you.

Set the intention that this crown will:

- Remind you to carry yourself with confidence
- Help others recognize your inherent worth
- Protect you from internalized shame or self-doubt
- Keep you centered in your own truth

This technique is especially useful before job interviews, family gatherings, or any situation where you might be tempted to diminish yourself to make others more comfortable.

Workplace Protection

For many LGBTQ+ people, the workplace presents unique challenges. Whether you're not out at work, dealing with subtle discrimination, or just trying to maintain professional relationships while being authentic, workplace protection magic can be incredibly helpful.

The Professional Glamour

Glamour, in magical terms, is about influencing how others perceive you. This technique helps you project competence, confidence, and authority while maintaining your authentic self.

What you need: A piece of jewelry or small object you can keep with you at work *Best time:* Before leaving for work or during your commute

Hold your chosen object and visualize it filling with

golden light. Set the intention that when you wear or carry this object, you will project:

- Professional competence and confidence
- Likability and trustworthiness
- Clear communication and leadership abilities
- Respect for your boundaries and identity

The key to effective glamour is that it enhances who you already are rather than creating a false persona. You're not trying to pretend to be someone else – you're simply making sure your best professional qualities shine through.

The Bathroom Mirror Blessing

For trans and gender non-conforming folks especially, workplace bathrooms can be a source of stress and vulnerability. This blessing helps create a sense of safety and belonging in these spaces.

When you're in a workplace bathroom (or any bathroom where you feel vulnerable), look at yourself in the mirror and silently say:

"I belong here. I am safe here. I am exactly who I'm meant to be. Any negative energy directed toward me bounces back to its source, transformed into understanding and compassion."

If looking in the mirror feels unsafe or uncomfortable, you can simply place your hand on your heart and speak these words internally.

Desk/Workspace Cleansing

Your workspace can accumulate negative energy from stress, conflict, and other people's emotions. Regular cleansing keeps your immediate environment clear and supportive.

What you need: Salt, a small bowl, or a cleansing spray (you can make one with water and a few drops of essential oil)

If you can use salt: Place a small amount in a bowl and keep it in your desk drawer or workspace. Replace it monthly, disposing of the old salt by flushing it down a toilet or throwing it away (not in a plant or outside, as you don't want to spread negative energy).

If salt isn't practical: Mix water with a few drops of lemon essential oil or peppermint oil in a small spray bottle. Once a week, lightly mist your workspace (test on a small area first to make sure it won't damage anything) while visualizing negative energy being dissolved and cleared away.

You can also cleanse energetically by simply visualizing white light filling your workspace and dissolving any heaviness or negativity.

Dating and Relationship Protection

Dating as a queer person comes with its own set of safety concerns. Beyond basic personal safety (which should always be your first priority), magical protection can help you navigate the emotional and energetic challenges of putting yourself out there.

First Date Safety Charm

What you need: A small object you can carry with you (a stone, piece of jewelry, or even a coin)

Before your date, hold the object and charge it with protective energy. Visualize it surrounded by white light and set the intention that it will:

- Help you accurately read the other person's energy and intentions
- Keep you grounded in your own truth and boundaries
- Attract honesty and authentic connection
- Protect you from deception or harmful intentions

Carry this object with you on the date. If at any point you feel uncomfortable or unsafe, hold the object and trust your intuition about whether to stay or leave.

Online Dating Profile Blessing

Before posting or updating your dating profile, perform this simple blessing to attract genuine connections while filtering out people who aren't right for you.

Place your hands on your phone or computer and visualize golden light flowing from your hands into your profile. Set the intention that your profile will:

- Attract people who will respect and value the real you
- Repel people who would waste your time or cause you harm
- Help you present your authentic self in the most appealing way
- Connect you with relationships that serve your highest good

Breakup Recovery Magic

Ending relationships is never easy, but it can be especially challenging when you're dealing with rejection related to your identity or when the queer dating pool feels limited.

Cord Cutting Ritual

What you need: Two candles, a piece of string or yarn, scissors, and a bowl of water

Light both candles and tie one end of the string to each candle (be careful not to create a fire hazard – the string should be taut but not touching the flames).

Visualize the string as representing the energetic connection between you and your ex. Hold the scissors and say:

"I release this connection with love and gratitude for what it taught me. I cut these ties so that we both may find happiness and healing. I am whole and complete on my own."

Cut the string and immediately drop the pieces into the bowl of water. Let the candles burn down safely (never leave them unattended), then dispose of the water and string pieces by pouring them down a drain.

Family Situations

Family can be one of the most challenging areas for LGBTQ+ folks, whether you're dealing with outright rejection, subtle disapproval, or the stress of not being out to family members. These protections can help you maintain your emotional equilibrium during difficult family interactions.

The Family Dinner Survival Kit

What you need: A small object you can keep in your pocket or bag

Before any potentially challenging family gathering, charge your chosen object with protective energy. Hold it and visualize it as a magical battery that stores:

- Confidence in your identity and worth
- Emotional stability and centeredness
- The ability to respond rather than react
- Connection to your chosen family and support system

During the gathering, touch or hold this object whenever you need to reconnect with your own truth and strength.

Boundary Setting Spell

This spell helps you maintain healthy boundaries with family members while staying open to love and connection where it's possible.

What you need: A white candle, a black candle, and a piece of paper

Write down the specific boundaries you want to maintain (e.g., "I will not discuss my transition with Uncle Bob," "I will leave if anyone uses slurs," "I will not justify my relationship to Mom").

Light the white candle and say: "I am open to love, respect, and healthy connection with my family."

Light the black candle and say: "I protect myself from harm, judgment, and disrespect. I am worthy of being treated with dignity."

Hold the paper between the two candles and say: "These boundaries serve love and truth. I maintain them with firmness and compassion."

Burn the paper safely and let both candles burn down completely.

Coming Out Protection

If you're planning to come out to family members, this protection ritual can help you feel more confident and centered.

What you need: A piece of rose quartz or another stone that feels supportive to you

Hold the stone and visualize it absorbing all your fears, worries, and doubts about coming out. Imagine these heavy emotions flowing out of your body and into the stone.

Now visualize the stone beginning to glow with warm, loving light. This light represents your courage, authenticity, and the love of everyone who already accepts you as you are.

Set the intention that this stone will remind you of your worth and help you speak your truth with confidence. Carry it with you when you come out, and hold it if you need courage or comfort.

TRAVEL PROTECTION

Whether you're traveling to a place with different cultural attitudes toward LGBTQ+ people or just want to feel safer while away from home, travel protection magic can provide peace of mind.

Safe Journey Blessing

Before you leave home, perform this blessing on your luggage, travel documents, and yourself.

Place your hands on your packed luggage and visualize protective white light surrounding it and everything in it. Set the intention that your belongings will be safe and that nothing you need will be lost or stolen.

Hold your travel documents and visualize them surrounded by golden light. Set the intention that your journey will be smooth and that you'll encounter helpful, friendly people along the way.

Finally, place your hands on your heart and say: "I travel safely and confidently. I am protected wherever I go. I attract kindness and respect from everyone I meet."

Hotel Room Cleansing

When you arrive at your accommodation, take a few minutes to clear and bless the space.

Walk around the room (including the bathroom) and visualize white light filling every corner, dissolving any negative energy left by previous occupants.

If you have salt with you, sprinkle a small amount in each corner of the room. If not, simply visualize protective light in each corner.

Set the intention that this space is now a sanctuary where you can rest safely and be completely yourself.

DIGITAL PROTECTION

Online harassment and privacy concerns are real issues for many LGBTQ+ people. While magical protection can't replace practical digital security measures, it can help protect your emotional well-being and energy in online spaces.

Social Media Shielding

Before opening social media apps, take a moment to visualize yourself surrounded by a bubble of protective light. Set the intention that:

- You will only see content that uplifts and informs you
- Negative comments and harassment will bounce off you without affecting your mood
- You will engage authentically but safely
- You will remember that online interactions don't define your worth

Email and Message Blessing

If you're expecting to receive potentially upsetting emails or messages (from family, work, dating apps, etc.), bless your inbox first.

Visualize your email or message inbox surrounded by filtering light that allows loving, respectful communication through while dissolving or blocking anything harmful.

Set the intention that you will receive the messages you need to see and that anything meant to hurt or upset you will lose its power before reaching you.

Emergency Protection

Sometimes we find ourselves in situations where we need immediate magical protection. These techniques can be done quickly and discretely in almost any circumstance.

The Instant Shield

Take a deep breath and visualize brilliant white light instantly surrounding your entire body. This light is impenetrable to negativity but transparent to love and respect.

Silently say: "I am safe, I am protected, I am exactly who I'm meant to be."

This entire technique takes less than 30 seconds and can be done anywhere.

The Mirror Technique

When someone is directing hostility, judgment, or negative energy toward you, visualize yourself as being made of mirrors. Their negativity bounces off you and returns to them, transformed into understanding and compassion.

This technique protects you from absorbing their negative energy while potentially helping them recognize their own behavior.

Calling in Support

In moments when you feel particularly vulnerable or alone, take a moment to energetically call in support from:

- Friends and chosen family who love you
- LGBTQ+ ancestors and elders who paved the way
- Your future self, who has navigated this challenge successfully
- Any spiritual guides or higher powers you work with

You don't have to face difficult situations alone. There's always a vast network of love and support available to you, both seen and unseen.

Making Protection Magic Your Own

Remember, the most effective protection magic is the kind that feels authentic and empowering to you. These techniques are starting points – feel free to modify them based on your own beliefs, needs, and circumstances.

Some people prefer to work with specific deities or guides for protection. Others like to incorporate crystals, herbs, or other tools. Some find that simple visualization is enough, while others need more elaborate rituals to feel confident in their magical work.

The key is consistency and belief. Regular protection

work becomes more effective over time as you build confidence in your own magical abilities and create strong energetic habits.

Most importantly, never let anyone tell you that you don't deserve protection, respect, and safety. Your magical practice should reinforce your inherent worth and help you move through the world with confidence and authenticity.

CHAPTER 3
Love Magic That Actually Works

Here's what most love spell books won't tell you: the best love magic starts with loving yourself. And as queer folks, we often have some extra work to do in that department.

Many of us grew up receiving messages that our desires, our identities, and our ways of loving were wrong. We might have spent years trying to fit into relationships that didn't honor who we really were. Some of us are still figuring out what healthy, authentic love looks like.

This chapter is about love magic that actually works – not because it forces someone to love you, but because it helps you become someone who attracts and maintains healthy, genuine connections. We'll start with self-love (yes, really), then move on to attracting authentic relationships, maintaining harmony with partners, and building chosen families.

The Daily Self-Love Check-In

This isn't a big ritual – just a simple practice you can do anywhere.

Once a day (maybe while brushing your teeth or drinking your morning coffee), put your hand on your heart and ask: "What do I need today to feel loved and supported?"

The answer might be:

- A compliment from yourself
- Permission to rest
- A text to a friend
- Time in nature
- Your favorite food
- A boundary with someone who drains your energy
- Celebrating a small accomplishment

Whatever comes up, try to honor that need if possible. This practice helps you become attuned to your own needs and teaches you that you can be a reliable source of love and care for yourself.

Mirror Work for Queer Folks

Mirror work can be challenging for anyone, but it can be especially complex for LGBTQ+ people who might have complicated relationships with their appearance or who are in the process of transitioning.

Start small and be gentle with yourself. Stand in front of a mirror and try to make eye contact with yourself. If that feels too intense, you can start by looking at your hands or another part of your body you feel neutral or positive about.

Say: "I am learning to love all of myself. I am worthy of respect and kindness, especially from me."

If full mirror work feels impossible right now, you can do this exercise by placing your hands on your heart and speaking to yourself with your eyes closed. The key is the intention to treat yourself with compassion, not the specific format.

The Identity Celebration Ritual

This ritual helps you honor and love all the aspects of your identity, including the parts that make you different or that others might not understand.

What you need: Colored candles or colored paper, and a few minutes of quiet time

Choose colors that represent different aspects of your identity. For example:

- Rainbow colors for your queer identity
- Pink, blue, and white for trans identity
- Colors that represent your cultural background, profession, hobbies, or other important parts of who you are

Light candles in these colors, or simply lay out colored paper in a pattern that feels meaningful to you.

For each color, say something like: "I celebrate and love this part of myself. This aspect of who I am is a gift, both to me and to the world."

Take time to really feel appreciation for the complexity and uniqueness of your identity. You're not just one thing – you're a whole constellation of wonderful qualities and experiences.

Transforming Shame into Power

Many LGBTQ+ folks carry shame about aspects of their identity or desires. This spell helps transform that shame into personal power.

What you need: A piece of paper, a pen, and a way to safely burn the paper (fireplace, cauldron, or metal bowl)

Write down any shame-based messages you've internalized about your identity, desires, or way of being. These might be things like:

- "There's something wrong with me"
- "I'm too much/not enough"
- "I don't deserve love"
- "My desires are shameful"

Don't spend too much time dwelling on these messages – just acknowledge them and write them down.

Now, on the other side of the paper, write the opposite – empowering truths about yourself:

- "I am exactly who I'm meant to be"
- "I am perfectly me"
- "I deserve love and respect"
- "My desires are natural and beautiful"

Hold the paper and say: "I release these old messages that never served me. I claim my power and my truth."

Burn the paper safely, visualizing the shame transforming into golden light that fills your heart with self-love and acceptance.

Attracting Authentic Connections

Now that we've laid the self-love foundation, let's talk about attracting relationships that actually fit your life. The key word here is "authentic" – we're not trying to manipulate anyone into loving us, but rather creating energetic conditions that help genuine connections flourish.

The Authentic Love Drawing Spell

This spell helps you attract romantic connections that honor all of who you are.

What you need: A pink or red candle, rose petals (fresh or dried), a piece of paper, and honey

Write down the qualities you want in a romantic partner, but focus on how you want to feel in the relationship rather than specific physical traits or circumstances. For example:

- "I want to feel seen and appreciated for who I really am"
- "I want to feel safe being vulnerable"
- "I want to laugh and have fun together"
- "I want to feel supported in my goals and dreams"
- "I want to feel sexually satisfied and desired"

Light the candle and sprinkle rose petals around it. Drizzle a small amount of honey on the paper (honey attracts sweetness and love) and say:

"I call to me a love that honors my authentic self. I attract someone who sees my beauty, celebrates my uniqueness, and loves me exactly as I am. This connection serves the highest good of all involved."

Fold the paper and keep it somewhere safe. Let the candle burn down completely.

The Dating App Blessing Ritual

Since many of us meet potential partners online, it makes sense to bring some magic to digital dating.

Before opening your dating app, hold your phone and visualize it surrounded by pink light. Set the intention that:

- You will attract matches who are genuinely interested in getting to know you
- You will easily recognize people who aren't right for you
- Your conversations will flow naturally and authentically

- You will feel confident and relaxed while dating

You can also "charge" your profile photos by visualizing them glowing with warm, attractive energy that draws in people who will appreciate your unique beauty and personality.

The Coffee Date Confidence Charm

First dates can be nerve-wracking, especially when you're not sure how the other person will react to your identity or when you're still figuring out if you want to be out to them.

What you need: A small object you can carry with you (stone, piece of jewelry, or coin)

Hold the object and charge it with confident, attractive energy. Visualize it glowing with golden light and set the intention that when you carry it:

- You will feel relaxed and confident
- Conversation will flow naturally
- You will accurately sense whether this person is right for you
- You will honor your own boundaries and needs
- The real you will shine through

Carry this charm on dates and touch it whenever you need to reconnect with your confidence.

Relationship Harmony Spells

Once you're in a relationship, different magical challenges arise. How do you maintain individual authenticity while building partnership? How do you work through conflicts constructively? How do you keep passion and connection alive as life gets complicated?

The Partnership Balance Ritual

This ritual is perfect for couples who want to maintain their individual identities while building a strong partnership.

What you need: Two candles (any color), a larger candle (white or yellow works well), and matches

You and your partner each light your own candle, representing your individual selves, dreams, and identities. Say something like:

"I honor who I am as an individual. I bring my whole self to this relationship, including my dreams, quirks, and needs."

Then together, use both your individual candles to light the larger candle, representing your partnership. Say together:

"We choose to build something beautiful together while remaining true to ourselves. Our love makes us both stronger and more authentic."

Let all three candles burn for a while (safely supervised), then blow out the individual candles while leaving the partnership candle burning. This symbolizes that while you're choosing to focus energy on your relationship, your individual selves remain intact and will be honored.

The Conflict Resolution Spell

Every relationship has conflicts, but this spell helps ensure they lead to greater understanding rather than lasting hurt.

What you need: A bowl of water, some salt, and a white candle

When you and your partner are having a disagreement, take a break from the conversation to perform this spell together (or you can do it alone if your partner isn't into magic).

Light the white candle and say: "We invite truth, compassion, and understanding into this situation."

Add a pinch of salt to the water and say: "We release the need to be right and open ourselves to being loving."

Both partners should dip their fingers in the salt water and touch their own hearts, then each other's hearts (with permission). Say together: "We speak from love and listen with love."

This ritual helps shift the energy from adversarial to collaborative, making it easier to find solutions that work for both of you.

Keeping Passion Alive

Long-term relationships can lose their spark, especially when life gets stressful. This spell helps rekindle passion and desire.

What you need: Red candles, cinnamon essential oil (or ground cinnamon), and something that represents your relationship (a photo, piece of jewelry you both wear, etc.)

Anoint the red candles with cinnamon oil or sprinkle them with ground cinnamon. Light them and place your relationship symbol between them.

Visualize the early days of your relationship – the excitement, attraction, and sense of possibility you felt. Let those feelings fill your heart, then imagine that energy flowing into your relationship symbol.

Say: "I choose to see my partner with fresh eyes. I choose to appreciate their beauty and uniqueness. I invite passion and playfulness back into our connection."

If you're doing this spell with your partner, take turns

sharing what you find attractive and exciting about each other. If you're doing it alone, focus on genuinely appreciating your partner's positive qualities and planning ways to express that appreciation.

Breakup Recovery Magic

Not all relationships last forever, and that's okay. Sometimes the most loving thing you can do is let a relationship end with grace and move forward with your heart open to new possibilities.

The Gratitude Release Ritual

This ritual helps you process the end of a relationship without getting stuck in bitterness or regret.
What you need: Two pieces of paper, a pen, and a way to safely burn paper

On one piece of paper, write everything you're grateful for about the relationship that's ending. Include lessons learned, happy memories, ways you grew, and anything positive you can honestly acknowledge.

On the second piece of paper, write everything you're ready to release – hurt feelings, expectations that weren't met, anger, disappointment, or hopes that won't be fulfilled.

Read both papers aloud, really feeling the emotions that come up. Then burn both papers safely, saying:

"I release this relationship with love and gratitude. I keep the lessons and let go of the pain. I am ready for whatever comes next."

Healing a Broken Heart

Heartbreak is especially complex for LGBTQ+ folks because the dating pool can feel limited, and rejection can trigger old wounds about being "too much" or not worthy of love.

What you need: Rose quartz or another heart-healing stone, green candles, and honey

Light green candles (for healing and new growth) and hold your rose quartz. Visualize your heart as cracked but not broken – like a beautiful mosaic that's being rebuilt with golden light.

Drizzle honey on your fingers and touch your heart, saying: "I am healing. I am worthy of love. This pain is temporary, but my capacity for love is eternal."

Carry the rose quartz with you for as long as you need the extra heart support.

Opening to Love Again

When you're ready to date again after a difficult breakup, this spell helps you open your heart while maintaining the wisdom you've gained.

What you need: A pink candle, a key (any kind), and a small mirror

Light the pink candle and hold the key, saying: "I hold the key to my own heart. I choose when to open it and to whom."

Look at yourself in the mirror and say: "I have learned and grown. I am ready to love and be loved again, with wisdom and joy."

Place the key somewhere special as a reminder that you control your own heart and that you can choose to be open to love while maintaining healthy boundaries.

Building Chosen Family

For many LGBTQ+ folks, chosen family is just as important as romantic relationships. These are the friends who become siblings, the mentors who become parental figures, and the community members who show up for all of life's big moments.

The Chosen Family Attraction Spell

This spell helps you attract the kind of deep, supportive friendships that become chosen family.
What you need: Orange candles (for friendship and community), a group photo or image that represents the kind of community you want, and cinnamon (for attraction)
Light the orange candles and place your image between them. Sprinkle cinnamon around the image and say:
"I call to me soul family – people who see and celebrate my true self. I attract friends who become chosen family, supporters who become lifelong companions. I am ready to give and receive this deep, authentic love."
Visualize yourself surrounded by loving, supportive people who truly get you. Feel the warmth and security of belonging to a community that celebrates your authentic self.

The Found Family Blessing

When you want to honor and strengthen the chosen family relationships you already have:
What you need: Photos of your chosen family members or objects that represent them
Arrange the photos or objects in a circle and light a candle in the center. Say:
"I bless these connections that nurture my soul. I am grateful for each person who chooses to love and support me. May our bonds grow stronger with time, and may I be as good a friend to them as they are to me."

Take a moment to send loving energy to each person represented, imagining your love reaching them wherever they are.

Community Building Magic

If you want to build stronger LGBTQ+ community in your area:
What you need: A yellow candle (for community and communication) and a map of your area
Light the yellow candle and place it on the map over your location. Say:
"I call together the queer folks in my area who are ready for authentic community. I attract people who want to support each other, celebrate together, and create chosen family bonds. May we find each other easily and build something beautiful together."
Visualize golden light spreading out from your location, connecting you with like-minded people in your area.

Dealing with Rejection and Discrimination

Unfortunately, LGBTQ+ folks often face rejection based on identity rather than compatibility. This section provides magical tools for processing this specific kind of hurt and moving forward with confidence.

The Rejection Transformation Spell

When someone rejects you because of your identity:
What you need: A black candle (for banishing negativity) and a white candle (for clarity and healing)
Light both candles and say:
"Their rejection is not a reflection of my worth. I transform this hurt into wisdom, this disappointment into discernment. I release any internalized shame and

remember that I deserve to be loved exactly as I am."

Let both candles burn down completely, visualizing the rejection losing its power to hurt you and transforming into protective wisdom that helps you recognize truly compatible people more quickly.

The Identity Affirmation Love Spell

This spell reinforces that your identity is not something to be tolerated in relationships – it's something to be celebrated.

What you need: Colored candles that represent your identity (rainbow, trans colors, etc.) and a mirror

Light your identity candles and look at yourself in the mirror. Say:

"My queerness is not a flaw to be overlooked – it's a gift that makes me who I am. I attract partners who don't just accept my identity but celebrate it. I deserve to be loved for my whole self, not in spite of parts of myself."

Feel the truth of these words sinking into your heart. You're not asking anyone to do you a favor by loving you – you're offering the gift of your authentic self to someone who's wise enough to recognize its value.

LOVE MAGIC ETHICS

Working love magic raises important questions about consent, free will, and ethics. Here are some guidelines that work well for queer practitioners:

Focus on yourself first.

The most effective and ethical love magic works on your own energy, confidence, and ability to attract healthy relationships rather than trying to make specific people fall in love with you.

Avoid targeting specific individuals.

Magic that tries to override someone's free will is generally not a good idea and often backfires anyway. Focus on attracting the right type of person rather than making a particular person love you.

Work for the highest good of all.

Include this phrase in your love spells to ensure that any magical results serve everyone involved, not just your immediate desires.

Remember that "no" is a complete sentence.

If someone isn't interested in you, respect that completely. Magic should never be used to overcome clear rejection or boundary-setting.

Consider harm carefully.

Ask yourself whether your magical goals could potentially hurt anyone (including yourself). If you're not sure, err on the side of caution.

Making Love Magic Part of Your Life

The most effective love magic becomes part of your daily life rather than something you only do during elaborate rituals. Here are some ways to incorporate love magic into regular routines:

Morning self-love affirmations while you get ready for the day

Gratitude practices that include appreciation for current relationships

Evening visualization where you imagine yourself surrounded by loving, supportive people

Regular cleansing of your living space to keep energy fresh and welcoming

Blessing your dates and social activities to attract positive connections

Remember, love magic isn't about desperation or forcing outcomes. It's about becoming the most authentic, confident version of yourself and creating energetic conditions that help genuine connections flourish. When you're radiating self-love and authenticity, you naturally attract people who appreciate and celebrate who you really are.

The best love magic helps you remember something you might have forgotten: you're inherently lovable, exactly as you are. Your queerness isn't something that makes you harder to love – it's part of what makes you beautifully, uniquely you.

CHAPTER 4
Career and Money Magic

Let's talk about something that affects all of us but that mainstream magical books often ignore: the intersection of career success, financial stability, and living authentically as LGBTQ+ people.

Many of us face unique challenges in the workplace – from outright discrimination to the exhausting decision of whether to come out in professional settings. Some of us work in industries where being openly queer could hurt our careers. Others struggle with imposter syndrome or internalized messages that we don't deserve success.

Then there's the financial piece. LGBTQ+ folks often face economic challenges related to family rejection, employment discrimination, or the additional costs that come with things like transition-related healthcare. Many of us also feel called to work that serves our communities, which might not always be the most financially lucrative path.

This chapter is about magical approaches to career and money that honor your authentic self while helping you build the financial security and professional satisfaction you deserve.

SHIFTING YOUR MONEY MINDSET

Before we get into specific spells, let's address something

crucial: your relationship with money itself. Many people have complicated feelings about money, but LGBTQ+ folks often carry additional layers of financial shame, fear, or confusion.

Maybe you grew up hearing that wanting money is shallow or selfish. Maybe you've internalized the idea that being different means you don't deserve the same opportunities as everyone else. Maybe you've been told that following your authentic path means accepting financial struggle.

Here's the truth: you deserve financial security. You deserve to be paid well for your work. You deserve to live comfortably and to have enough money to support the causes and communities you care about. Your queerness doesn't make you less deserving of abundance – it gives you unique perspectives and skills that add value to the world.

The Abundance Affirmation Practice

Every morning for a week, before you check your bank account, pay bills, or think about money stress, spend five minutes doing this practice:

Place your hand on your heart and say: "I deserve financial security and abundance. My unique gifts and perspectives are valuable. I attract opportunities that honor my authentic self while providing financial stability. Money flows to me easily and I use it wisely."

Notice any resistance that comes up – thoughts like "that's not realistic" or "people like me don't get those opportunities." Don't fight these thoughts, just acknowledge them and return to the affirmation.

The Money Story Rewrite

What you need: Paper, pen, and a way to safely burn the

paper

Write down all the negative messages you've internalized about money, especially as they relate to your identity. These might include:

- "Queer people can't be successful in mainstream careers"
- "Following your authentic path means being broke"
- "Wanting money is shallow"
- "People like me don't deserve wealth"
- "I have to choose between being authentic and being financially secure"

Read through what you've written, then on a new piece of paper, rewrite each statement as an empowering truth:

- "My queer perspective is an asset in any career"
- "Authenticity attracts the right opportunities"
- "Wanting financial security is wise and healthy"
- "I deserve abundance as much as anyone"
- "I can be fully authentic and financially successful"

Burn the old messages and keep the new ones somewhere you'll see them regularly.

JOB SEARCH MAGIC

Looking for work can be stressful for anyone, but LGBTQ+ folks often have additional concerns: Will this workplace be safe? Should I come out in interviews? How do I handle gaps in my resume related to transition or coming out? Can I be authentic and still get hired?

The Right Opportunity Attraction Spell

This spell helps you attract job opportunities that are

genuinely good fits – places where you can be successful, authentic, and valued.

What you need: Green candles (for prosperity and growth), bay leaves, and a pen

Write your ideal job qualities on bay leaves. Focus on the work environment and how you want to feel rather than specific job titles or companies:

- "I feel respected and valued for my unique contributions"
- "I work with people who appreciate diversity"
- "I feel safe being my authentic self"
- "I am paid fairly for my skills and experience"
- "I have opportunities for growth and advancement"

Light the green candles and burn the bay leaves safely, visualizing the smoke carrying your intentions out into the universe.

Say: "I attract work opportunities that serve my highest good. The right job finds me easily, and I recognize it when it appears."

Resume Blessing Ritual

Before sending out your resume, perform this blessing to ensure it reaches the right people and makes a positive impression.

What you need: Your resume (printed or on your computer screen), frankincense or another success-drawing incense, and gold or yellow light (candle or visualization)

Light the incense and hold your hands over your resume. Visualize golden light flowing from your hands into the document.

Say: "This resume accurately represents my skills and value. It reaches the right people at the right time and creates opportunities for authentic, fulfilling work."

If you're concerned about gaps in your resume or other challenges related to your identity, visualize those concerns dissolving in the golden light, replaced by confidence in your overall qualifications and unique perspective.

Interview Confidence Charm

What you need: A small piece of citrine, carnelian, or another confidence-boosting stone (or any small object that feels empowering to you)

Hold the stone and charge it with confident, professional energy. Visualize it glowing with golden light and set the intention that when you carry it:

- You feel calm and confident
- Your best professional qualities shine through
- You communicate clearly and authentically
- You accurately assess whether this opportunity is right for you
- The interviewer remembers you positively

Carry this charm to interviews and hold it whenever you need to reconnect with your confidence.

Workplace Success Magic

Once you have a job, different magical challenges arise. How do you navigate workplace politics while staying authentic? How do you build professional relationships when you're not fully out? How do you advance in your career while maintaining your integrity?

The Professional Authenticity Balance

This ongoing magical practice helps you find the right balance between professional success and authentic self-expression.

Each morning before work, take a moment to visualize yourself surrounded by a professional glamour – not a fake persona, but the most confident, competent version of your authentic self.

Set the daily intention: "I bring my whole self to work while adapting appropriately to professional situations. I find ways to be authentic that serve both my career and my integrity."

Throughout the day, when you face decisions about how much of yourself to share or how to respond to various situations, check in with this intention and trust your intuition about the right balance for each moment.

The Promotion Manifestation Spell

When you're ready for career advancement:
What you need: A green candle, a piece of paper, and cinnamon (for success and attraction)

Write down the promotion, raise, or career advancement you want, including:

- The type of role or responsibilities you want
- The salary range you're targeting
- The timeline you're hoping for
- How this advancement will serve your larger goals

Sprinkle cinnamon on the paper, light the green candle, and say:

"I am ready for greater responsibility and recognition. My skills, perspective, and hard work deserve advancement. Opportunities for growth come to me easily, and I recognize and seize them confidently."

Fold the paper and keep it in your wallet or workspace. Take concrete actions toward your goal while trusting that magical energy is supporting your efforts.

Workplace Discrimination Protection

Unfortunately, workplace discrimination is still a reality for many LGBTQ+ folks. While magic can't replace legal protections or HR policies, it can help you navigate these challenges with greater strength and clarity.

What you need: Black tourmaline or another protective stone, white sage or cleansing incense

Cleanse your protective stone with the sage smoke and charge it with protective energy. Set the intention that this stone will:

- Help you recognize discrimination clearly without second-guessing yourself
- Keep you grounded and professional in difficult situations
- Attract allies and support when you need them
- Protect you from absorbing others' negative energy
- Guide you toward appropriate responses and resources

Carry this stone at work and hold it whenever you need extra strength or clarity.

ENTREPRENEURSHIP AND CREATIVE WORK MAGIC

Many LGBTQ+ folks are drawn to entrepreneurship or creative work, either because we want the freedom to be fully authentic or because we want to serve our communities. But starting a business or pursuing creative work comes with its own financial and professional challenges.

The Creative Block Breaker

When you're stuck on a project or struggling with

creative inspiration:

What you need: Orange candles (for creativity and inspiration), fresh flowers or plants, and your creative tools (computer, paints, instruments, etc.)

Arrange the flowers around your workspace and light the orange candles. Hold your hands over your creative tools and say:

"I am a channel for creative inspiration. Ideas flow through me easily and joyfully. I trust my creative instincts and express them boldly."

Work on your project for at least 15 minutes, even if you don't feel particularly inspired when you start. Often, the act of beginning is enough to get creative energy flowing again.

The Client Attraction Spell

For freelancers, consultants, and small business owners who need to attract ideal clients:

What you need: Gold or green candles, a business card or something that represents your services, and honey

Place your business card between the candles and drizzle it lightly with honey (for attraction and sweetness). Light the candles and say:

"I attract clients who value my work and pay me fairly. My ideal clients find me easily and recognize the value I provide. Working together serves the highest good of all involved."

Visualize your calendar filling up with work from clients who appreciate your unique perspective and pay you well for your expertise.

The Side Hustle Success Ritual

Many people need side hustles for extra income, and this

can be especially true for LGBTQ+ folks who might face employment discrimination or want to build financial independence.

What you need: Two green candles and a coin or piece of currency

Light both candles and hold the coin between them. Visualize the coin multiplying – first into two coins, then four, then more and more.

Say: "This side income grows steadily and sustainably. I attract opportunities that fit my schedule and skills. This additional money provides security and freedom."

Keep the coin in your wallet as a reminder of your growing abundance.

FINANCIAL HEALING AND ABUNDANCE

Many of us carry financial trauma from family rejection, employment discrimination, or simply growing up with limited resources. Healing these wounds is crucial for building sustainable abundance.

The Financial Trauma Healing Ritual

What you need: Blue candles (for healing), a bowl of salt water, and a soft cloth

Light the blue candles and dip your fingers in the salt water. Touch your heart and say:

"I release old fears and wounds around money. I heal from past financial trauma and open myself to abundance. I deserve security, comfort, and the freedom that financial stability provides."

Use the soft cloth to gently dry your fingers, symbolizing the gentle care you're giving yourself as you heal.

The Gratitude Abundance Practice

This daily practice helps shift your focus from scarcity to abundance: Every evening, write down three things you're financially grateful for that day. These can be small things:

- "I had enough money for lunch"
- "My paycheck deposited on time"
- "A friend bought me coffee"
- "I found a quarter on the sidewalk"

This practice trains your brain to notice abundance that's already present in your life, which makes it easier to attract more.

The Emergency Fund Spell

Building an emergency fund is crucial for financial security, especially for LGBTQ+ folks who might face unexpected discrimination or family issues.

What you need: A jar or container, green paper or cloth, and any amount of money (even a dollar bill or some coins)

Wrap your container in green paper or cloth and place the money inside. Each week, add whatever amount you can, even if it's just pocket change.

As you add money, say: "This fund grows steadily and provides security. I always have enough for emergencies and unexpected opportunities."

The key is consistency, not the amount. Even adding a dollar a week creates momentum and magical energy around financial security.

Career Transition Magic

Sometimes we need to make major career changes – either because our current work doesn't fit our authentic selves or because we want to pursue something more meaningful. Career transitions can be scary, especially when you're already navigating other aspects of identity and belonging.

The Career Transition Clarity Ritual

When you're considering a career change but aren't sure what direction to go:
What you need: White candles (for clarity), a journal, and quiet time
Light the white candles and ask yourself these questions, writing down whatever comes up without censoring:

- What kind of work energizes me?
- What problems do I love solving?
- What would I do if money wasn't a concern?
- What careers would allow me to be fully authentic?
- What skills do I have that I'm not currently using?
- What kind of impact do I want to have?

Don't worry about being practical at this stage – just let your authentic desires emerge. You can figure out the practical steps later.

The Bridge Building Spell

When you know what career direction you want but aren't sure how to get there:
What you need: Two candles (any color), a piece of string or ribbon, and small objects that represent your current situation and your goal
Place one candle and one object at each end of your workspace. Tie one end of the string to each object, creating a bridge between them.

Light both candles and say: "I build a bridge between where I am and where I want to be. The path becomes clear, and I take one step at a time with confidence."

Over the coming weeks, pay attention to opportunities, connections, and ideas that could help you move toward your goal. Often, the "bridge" appears in the form of small, practical steps rather than one dramatic change.

Money Magic Ethics

Working money magic raises questions about fairness, greed, and social responsibility. Here are some guidelines that work well for LGBTQ+ practitioners:

Consider the source.

Money magic works by attracting opportunities, not by taking resources away from others. Focus on creating value and expanding possibilities rather than taking from a limited pie.

Remember your values.

Include intentions about using money in ways that align with your values – supporting causes you care about, helping your community, living sustainably, etc.

Stay grounded.

Money magic should complement practical actions like skill-building, networking, and smart financial planning, not replace them.

Share your abundance.

As your financial situation improves, find ways to

support others – whether that's through formal charitable giving, mutual aid, or simply being generous with friends who are struggling.

INTEGRATING CAREER AND MONEY MAGIC INTO DAILY LIFE

The most effective career and money magic becomes part of your regular routine rather than something you only do during formal spells. Here are some ways to maintain magical momentum:

Morning abundance affirmations while you get ready for work

Blessing your paycheck when it arrives, even if it's smaller than you'd like

Visualizing career success during your commute

Cleansing your workspace regularly to keep energy flowing

Gratitude practices that include appreciation for your skills and opportunities

Setting weekly intentions about career and financial goals

The Bigger Picture

Remember, career and money magic isn't just about personal success – it's about claiming your right to participate fully in economic life as an authentic LGBTQ+ person. Every time you advance in your career while staying true to yourself, you're opening doors for others. Every time you build financial security, you're creating stability that allows you to support your community and causes you care about.

Your success matters, not just for you but for all the young LGBTQ+ people who need to see that it's possible to be authentic and prosperous, to follow your dreams and pay your bills, to be proudly queer and professionally successful.

The world needs what you have to offer. Magic can help you claim the career satisfaction and financial security that allow you to offer it fully.

CHAPTER 5
Gender Magic and Body Blessings

Gender is one of the most fundamentally magical aspects of human experience – it's about identity, transformation, self-determination, and the power to define yourself on your own terms. For many LGBTQ+ folks, especially transgender and gender non-conforming people, gender is already a conscious, intentional practice rather than something that just happens automatically.

This chapter is for anyone whose relationship with gender is complex, evolving, or outside the mainstream. Whether you're transitioning, questioning, non-binary, or simply want a different relationship with your body and gender expression, these magical practices can support your journey toward authenticity and self-love.

Gender as Magic, Magic as Gender

Think about it: gender transition is literally transformation magic. It's about envisioning who you really are, setting intentions for how you want to be seen and experienced in the world, and then taking concrete steps to make that vision reality. It's about the power of naming yourself, choosing your own pronouns, and insisting that the world recognize your truth.

Non-binary and genderfluid experiences are also inherently magical – they require holding multiple truths simultaneously, being comfortable with change and ambiguity, and creating new possibilities outside existing categories. These are all fundamentally magical skills.

Even cisgender folks who want to explore different aspects of gender expression, or who want to heal from restrictive gender messaging, are engaging in gender magic when they consciously choose how to embody and express their gender.

Affirming Your Authentic Self

The foundation of all gender magic is the radical act of affirming who you really are, regardless of what others might think or expect.

The Daily Identity Affirmation

This practice can be done anywhere – in the mirror, during your commute, or even silently during challenging social situations.

Place your hand on your heart (or touch a piece of jewelry, or simply focus inward if touching isn't possible) and silently or quietly say:

"I am exactly who I'm meant to be. My gender identity is valid and beautiful. I deserve to be seen, respected, and celebrated for who I really am."

If you're in the process of transitioning or exploring your gender, you might say:

"I am becoming more myself every day. I trust my inner knowing about who I am. I have the right to express my authentic gender."

For non-binary folks:

"I don't need to fit into someone else's categories. My gender is valid even if others don't understand it. I define myself."

The Name Blessing Ritual

Whether you're choosing a new name, adding a middle name, or simply want to bless the name you already have, this ritual honors the power of naming yourself.

What you need: A white candle, a piece of paper, and a pen

Write your name (whatever name feels most authentic to you right now) on the paper. This might be a legal name, chosen name, nickname, or even a private name you're still exploring.

Light the white candle and hold the paper. Say:

"This name holds my essence and my truth. When this name is spoken with respect, it honors all of who I am. I claim this name and all the power it holds."

If you're in the process of changing your name socially or legally, you can modify this to:

"I release my old name with gratitude for how it served me. I claim my new name and all the possibilities it represents. I am reborn into my truth."

Keep the paper somewhere safe as a reminder of your self-determination and power.

Pronoun Protection Spells

For many people, using correct pronouns is a basic sign of respect, but for trans and non-binary folks, pronouns can be a source of both affirmation and stress. These spells help create energetic support around pronoun usage.

The Pronoun Shield

This visualization can be done anywhere and helps protect you from the emotional impact of being misgendered.

When you're entering a situation where you might be misgendered, visualize your correct pronouns written in golden light around your body. See them glowing brightly, reminding everyone you encounter of your true identity.

Set the intention: "My pronouns are clear and visible to those who are ready to see me. When someone uses incorrect pronouns, it reflects their limitations, not my reality."

This doesn't magically make everyone use correct pronouns, but it can help you feel more centered and confident, and some people report that others do seem to use correct pronouns more often.

The Pronoun Blessing for Allies

If you're an ally who wants to support the trans and non-binary people in your life, this spell can help you remember and use correct pronouns consistently.

What you need: A small notebook or your phone's notes app

Write down the correct pronouns for each trans or non-binary person in your life. Hold the list and say:

"I commit to seeing and honoring each person's true identity. I remember their pronouns easily and use them naturally. My words reflect my respect for who they really are."

Review this list regularly until using correct pronouns becomes automatic.

Recovery from Misgendering

When you've been misgendered and need to process the emotional impact:

What you need: A bowl of cool water and a soft towel

Dip your hands in the cool water and place them on your heart. Say:

"Other people's words cannot change who I am. I wash away the sting of their misunderstanding and reconnect with my own truth. I am who I know myself to be."

Dry your hands gently with the towel, symbolizing the care you're giving yourself.

TRANSITION SUPPORT MAGIC

Transitioning – whether social, medical, or legal – is already a magical process of transformation. These spells can provide additional energetic support for various aspects of transition.

The Transition Timeline Blessing

This spell helps you trust the timing of your transition process, especially when it feels like things are moving too slowly or when you're facing delays with medical care, legal documents, or other practical aspects.

What you need: A calendar or journal, green candles (for growth and patience), and a pen

Light the green candles and look at your calendar. Mark important transition milestones – past, present, and future. These might include:

- First time you used your chosen name
- Coming out to important people
- Starting hormones
- Scheduled surgeries
- Legal name change appointments
- Any other significant markers

Say: "I trust the timing of my journey. Each step happens when it's meant to happen. I am patient with the process while staying committed to my goals."

This helps you see transition as an ongoing journey rather than a destination, and can provide comfort during waiting periods.

The Medical Transition Support Spell

For those pursuing medical transition (hormones, surgeries, etc.):

What you need: Blue candles (for healing), a photo of yourself that you love, and any medical transition supplies you're currently using

Light the blue candles and place your photo between them. Hold your transition supplies (hormone bottles, compression garments, etc.) and say:

"I bless this journey of aligning my body with my truth. I trust my medical team and my own wisdom about what's right for me. My body is becoming a truer expression of who I am."

Visualize golden healing light surrounding your body and supporting all the changes you're making.

The Social Transition Courage Spell

Coming out and living openly in your authentic gender takes courage, especially in new environments or with people you're not sure will be supportive.

What you need: A piece of citrine or carnelian (for courage), or any small object that makes you feel brave

Hold the object and charge it with courageous energy. Visualize it glowing with bright, confident light and set the intention that when you carry it:

- You feel calm and confident about being yourself
- You attract accepting, supportive people
- You have the strength to handle any negativity gracefully
- You remember that your authenticity is a gift, not a burden

Carry this courage charm when you're coming out to new people or navigating challenging social situations.

BODY RELATIONSHIP MAGIC

Many LGBTQ+ folks have complex relationships with their bodies – whether due to gender dysphoria, body image issues related to not fitting societal norms, or simply the challenge of loving a body in a world that sends so many negative messages about difference.

The Body Gratitude Practice

This practice helps you develop a more loving relationship with your body, even if that relationship feels complicated right now.

Each day, find one thing about your body that you can genuinely appreciate. This doesn't have to be appearance-related – it can be functional:

- "Thank you, hands, for creating beautiful things"
- "Thank you, legs, for carrying me where I need to go"
- "Thank you, voice, for letting me speak my truth"
- "Thank you, heart, for keeping me alive"

If you're dealing with significant body dysphoria, you might need to start very small:

- "Thank you, lungs, for breathing automatically"
- "Thank you, body, for healing from cuts and bruises"

The goal is to gradually shift from seeing your body as an enemy to seeing it as an ally in living your authentic life.

The Dysphoria Soothing Ritual

For times when gender dysphoria feels overwhelming:
What you need: Lavender essential oil (or any scent that feels calming to you), a soft blanket or comfortable clothing

Apply a small amount of lavender oil to your wrists or chest (test on a small area first to make sure you're not sensitive). Wrap yourself in the soft blanket or change into comfortable clothing.

Take slow, deep breaths and say:

"This discomfort is part of my journey. My body is a work in progress, and I honor its changes. I give myself the grace to heal and grow."

Instead of focusing on eliminating the dysphoria, prioritize grounding yourself. Try a simple activity like tracing your fingers along the blanket's texture, listening to calming music, or visualizing a place where you feel safe and whole. Let yourself feel supported in this moment.

The Mirror Work for Gender Affirmation

Mirror work can be particularly challenging for people with complicated relationships with their appearance, but it can also be powerfully healing when approached gently.

Start by looking at yourself in the mirror for just a few

seconds. If that feels too intense, start by looking at your hands or another part of your body you feel neutral about.

Say: "I see someone who is brave enough to live authentically. I see someone who is constantly growing and becoming. I am learning to love what I see."

If full mirror work feels impossible, you can do this by placing your hands on your heart and speaking to yourself with your eyes closed.

BINDING AND UNBINDING SPELLS

These spells are metaphorical and energetic – they're about releasing restrictions and claiming freedom to express yourself authentically.

The Restriction Release Ritual

This spell helps you release internalized messages about how you "should" express your gender.

What you need: A piece of string or ribbon, scissors, and a white candle

Light the white candle and loosely tie the string around your wrist (not tightly – this should be comfortable and easy to remove).

Think about all the messages you've received about how you should look, act, dress, or express your gender. Say:

"I release all expectations that don't serve my authentic self. I cut the ties that bind me to others' ideas about who I should be."

Cut the string and let it fall away, symbolizing your freedom from restrictive gender expectations.

The Expression Liberation Spell

This spell supports you in expressing your gender more freely and authentically.

What you need: Colored ribbons, scarves, or fabric that represent how you want to express your gender, and a mirror

Drape the fabric around yourself in whatever way feels good – as clothing, accessories, or simply decoration. Look at yourself in the mirror and say:

"I claim my right to express my gender in whatever way feels authentic to me. I dress, move, and present myself in ways that honor my truth. My gender expression is beautiful and valid."

Take a few moments to appreciate how the colors and textures make you feel. Remember this feeling of authentic self-expression.

CLOTHING AND PRESENTATION MAGIC

What we wear and how we present ourselves to the world can be deeply magical, especially for people whose authentic gender expression might not match societal expectations.

The Wardrobe Blessing Ritual

Whether you're building a new wardrobe that matches your identity or want to bless the clothes you already own:

What you need: Your favorite piece of gender-affirming clothing and some lavender or rosemary (for blessing and protection)

Hold your clothing item and sprinkle it lightly with the herbs (brush them off afterward if needed). Say:

"I bless these clothes that help me express my authentic self. When I wear clothing that affirms my gender, I feel confident, comfortable, and true to who I am."

You can extend this blessing to your entire wardrobe by visualizing the same energy flowing to all your clothes.

The Confidence Glamour

This magical technique helps you project confidence and authenticity, especially when you're wearing clothing or presentation that's new or that might attract attention.

Before getting dressed, visualize golden light filling your body and radiating outward. Set the intention that this light will:

- Help others see your confidence and authenticity
- Make your chosen presentation look natural and right on you
- Deflect any negative judgments or stares
- Attract compliments and positive attention

As you get dressed, imagine each piece of clothing being charged with this confident, authentic energy.

The Outfit Armor Spell

For days when you need extra protection while expressing your gender authentically:

Choose your outfit with intention, picking pieces that make you feel strong and confident. As you put on each item, visualize it as a piece of magical armor that protects you while allowing your true self to shine through.

Say: "I armor myself with authenticity. My clothes express my truth and protect my spirit. I move through the world confidently and safely."

Bathroom and Changing Room Protection

These spaces can be particularly challenging for trans and gender non-conforming folks. While magic can't replace legal protections or policy changes, it can provide emotional and energetic support.

The Bathroom Blessing

Before entering a public restroom that makes you feel anxious:

Take a deep breath and visualize yourself surrounded by protective light. Say silently: "I belong here. I am safe here. I use the facilities I need with confidence and peace."

If someone challenges your presence, this visualization can help you stay calm and respond appropriately to the situation.

The Changing Room Confidence Charm

What you need: A small object you can carry with you (a stone, piece of jewelry, or coin)

Charge the object with confident, protective energy by holding it and visualizing it glowing with golden light. Set the intention that when you carry it into changing rooms or other vulnerable spaces, it will remind you of your right to exist and take up space.

The "I Belong Here" Mantra

This simple mantra can be used in any space where your presence might be questioned:

Silently repeat: "I belong here. I have every right to be here. I am exactly where I need to be."

Focus on your breathing and your right to exist in public spaces as your authentic self.

HONORING YOUR GENDER JOURNEY

Your relationship with gender is unique, and it may continue to evolve throughout your life. These practices help you honor that journey and stay connected to your authentic self as you grow and change.

The Gender Timeline Ritual

This ritual helps you honor all the stages of your gender journey – past, present, and future.

What you need: Colored candles or paper representing different stages of your gender experience, and a journal

Light candles or lay out colored paper to represent different phases of your gender journey. For each phase, write or speak about:

- What you learned during that time
- How that experience shaped who you are today
- What you're grateful for from that period
- How you've grown and changed

End by lighting a special candle or choosing a special color for your current self and your future growth.

The Chosen Family Gender Blessing

If you have friends or chosen family who've supported your gender journey:

What you need: Photos of supportive people or objects that represent them

Arrange the photos or objects and light a candle for each person. Say:

"I am grateful for the people who see and celebrate my authentic gender. I am blessed by chosen family who use my correct name and pronouns, who support my journey, and who love me exactly as I am."

Send loving energy to each person, thanking them for their support and acceptance.

Creating Sacred Gender Space

Whether you live alone or with others, it's important to have spaces where you can express your gender freely and authentically.

The Sacred Space Gender Blessing

Choose a space in your home that can be dedicated to authentic gender expression – this might be your bedroom, a corner of a room, or even just a drawer or box where you keep special items.

What you need: Items that represent your authentic gender (clothing, photos, jewelry, colors, symbols, etc.)

Arrange these items in your chosen space and say:

"This space honors my authentic gender. Here I am free to explore, express, and celebrate all aspects of who I am. This space holds my truth and supports my journey."

Visit this space whenever you need to reconnect with your authentic self or when you're preparing for challenging situations.

The Mirror Altar

Create a small altar space around a mirror where you can practice gender affirmation and self-love.

Include:

- Photos of yourself that you love
- Items in colors that represent your gender identity
- Affirming notes or quotes
- Small objects that make you feel confident and authentic

Use this space for daily affirmations, getting ready for important events, or whenever you need to reconnect with your authentic self.

Gender Magic for Allies

If you're a cisgender person who wants to support the trans and gender non-conforming people in your life, magic can help you be a better ally.

The Ally Education Spell

What you need: A purple candle (for wisdom and understanding) and a journal

Light the purple candle and ask for guidance in understanding gender experiences different from your own. Write down questions you have, and commit to seeking out educational resources created by trans and gender non-conforming people themselves.

Say: "I open my mind and heart to understanding experiences different from my own. I educate myself so I can be a better ally and advocate."

The Pronoun Respect Ritual

What you need: A piece of paper with the correct pronouns for each trans or gender non-conforming person in your life

Hold the paper and say: "I commit to honoring each person's gender identity through my words and actions. I practice using correct pronouns until it becomes natural. My respect is demonstrated through consistent, accurate language."

Practice using the pronouns out loud until they flow naturally.

Integration and Daily Practice

Gender magic works best when it's integrated into your daily life rather than reserved for special occasions. Here are some ways to maintain magical momentum:

Morning gender affirmations as part of your getting-ready routine

Blessing your clothes as you get dressed each day

Gratitude for your body even if the relationship is complicated

Pronoun meditation when you need to center yourself in your identity

Protective visualization before entering potentially challenging spaces

Evening appreciation for moments when you felt authentically yourself

The Bigger Picture

Remember that your gender magic isn't just personal – it's political. Every time you live authentically as a trans or gender non-conforming person, you're making it easier for others to do the same. Every time you insist on being seen and respected for who you are, you're expanding possibilities for future generations.

Your authenticity is revolutionary. Your existence is resistance. And your magic – the daily practice of becoming more yourself, of insisting on your right to define yourself, of transforming both your own life and the world around you – that magic matters more than you might realize.

The world needs people who understand that gender is creative, fluid, and self-determined. Your magic contributes to a future where all people can express their authentic gender freely and safely.

CHAPTER 6
Community and Celebration Magic

One of the most beautiful aspects of LGBTQ+ life is the way we create community and celebration out of necessity, joy, and shared experience. We gather to celebrate Pride, to mark personal milestones, to honor those we've lost, and to create chosen families that sustain us through all of life's challenges.

This chapter is about magical practices that strengthen community bonds, enhance celebrations, and help create the kind of inclusive, loving spaces where everyone can show up authentically. Whether you're planning a Pride event, celebrating a friend's transition milestone, or simply wanting to create more magical community in your daily life, these practices can help.

PRIDE MAGIC AND SEASONAL CELEBRATIONS

Pride season is inherently magical – it's about transformation, visibility, celebration, and community power. But you don't have to wait for June to bring Pride energy into your life.

The Pride Altar Creation

Create a magical space that honors both your personal Pride journey and the broader LGBTQ+ community.

What you need: Rainbow colors (candles, fabric, flowers, or paper), photos of LGBTQ+ ancestors and elders, and items that represent your own journey

Arrange your rainbow colors in whatever pattern feels right to you – this might be the traditional Pride flag order, or you might include additional colors like the trans Pride flag, Bear Pride flag, or other identity flags that represent your community.

Add photos or symbols representing LGBTQ+ people who've paved the way – this might include famous activists, but also friends, mentors, or community members who've influenced your journey.

Include something personal: a photo from your first Pride, a piece of jewelry that represents your identity, or any object that connects you to your authentic self.

Light candles and say: "I honor all who came before me, all who stand with me now, and all who will follow. I am part of a beautiful, diverse, powerful community. My pride in who I am contributes to our collective strength."

The Year-Round Pride Practice

Pride doesn't have to be limited to one month. This daily practice helps you maintain Pride energy throughout the year.

Each morning, choose one thing about your LGBTQ+ identity that you're genuinely proud of. This might be:

- Your courage in living authentically
- Your ability to love in ways that don't fit narrow definitions
- Your resilience in facing challenges
- Your contribution to LGBTQ+ community
- Your growth in self-acceptance
- Your role in supporting other queer folks

Hold this feeling of pride as you start your day, and let it influence how you move through the world.

The Community Celebration Blessing

Before any LGBTQ+ celebration or gathering:
What you need: A group of people (this can be done with just one other person) and something to share (food, drink, or even just words)

Form a circle (or sit together if you're just two people) and pass around whatever you're sharing. As each person receives it, they share one thing they're grateful for about LGBTQ+ community.

End with everyone saying together: "We celebrate our authentic selves, our chosen families, and our powerful community. Our joy is resistance, our love is revolution, our presence is a gift to the world."

HONORING LGBTQ+ ANCESTORS AND ELDERS

Our community has a rich history of resilience, creativity, and activism. Honoring those who came before us strengthens our connection to this legacy and helps us remember that we're part of something larger than ourselves.

The Ancestor Appreciation Ritual

What you need: Purple candles (for honoring elders), photos or names of LGBTQ+ ancestors you want to honor, and flowers or another offering

This can include famous figures like Marsha P. Johnson, Sylvia Rivera, Harvey Milk, or Audre Lorde, but also personal mentors, friends who've passed away, or community elders who've influenced your life.

Light the purple candles and arrange your photos or write down names. Say:

"We remember those who fought for our freedom, who lived boldly when it was dangerous to do so, who created spaces where we could be ourselves. We honor their courage, their creativity, and their love. We commit to carrying their legacy forward."

Spend time thinking about specific ways these ancestors have influenced your life or the broader community. Leave the flowers as an offering and a symbol of your gratitude.

The Elder Wisdom Circle

If you have older LGBTQ+ folks in your community, create opportunities to learn from their experiences.

What you need: A comfortable gathering space and willingness to listen

Invite LGBTQ+ elders to share their stories – how they found community, what challenges they overcame, what advice they have for younger generations. Create a sacred space for these stories by:

- Opening with gratitude for their presence and wisdom
- Asking questions that honor their experiences
- Listening without trying to fix or judge
- Closing with appreciation for what they've shared

This isn't just about learning history – it's about strengthening intergenerational connections and ensuring that wisdom gets passed down.

The Daily Elder Blessing

Each day, take a moment to send loving energy to LGBTQ+ elders, both those you know personally and those in the broader community.

Say: "I send love and gratitude to the elders who paved the way for my freedom. I appreciate their sacrifices, their courage, and their ongoing wisdom. May they feel honored and supported by our community."

CREATING SACRED QUEER SPACE

Sometimes the most magical thing we can do is create spaces where LGBTQ+ folks can gather, connect, and be completely authentic. This might be in your home, at community events, or even online.

The Space Blessing Ritual

Before hosting any LGBTQ+ gathering:
What you need: Salt or another cleansing agent, rainbow colors (however you want to incorporate them), and a clear intention

Cleanse the space by sprinkling salt in the corners or burning cleansing incense. As you do this, set the intention that this space will be:

- Safe for all LGBTQ+ identities
- Free from judgment and discrimination
- Welcoming to people at all stages of their journey
- A place where authentic connections can form
- Protected from negative energy or harmful intentions

Incorporate rainbow colors through decorations, lighting, food, or simply visualization. Say:
"This space is blessed and sacred. All who enter are welcomed with love and acceptance. Here we can be our full, authentic selves without fear or shame."

The Community Circle Opening

For the beginning of LGBTQ+ group meetings, support groups, or social gatherings:

What you need: Participants willing to share briefly

Form a circle (physical or virtual) and have each person share:

- Their name and pronouns
- One word describing how they're feeling right now
- One thing they hope to give to or receive from the group

End with everyone saying together: "We create sacred space through our presence, our authenticity, and our commitment to supporting each other."

The Chosen Family Blessing

For groups that function as chosen family:

What you need: A candle for each person, and a larger central candle

Each person lights their individual candle from the central flame, saying: "I bring my authentic self to this chosen family."

When everyone's candle is lit, say together: "We choose each other. We support each other through joy and challenge. We celebrate each other's growth and hold each other in love. We are family by choice and commitment."

Let the candles burn for a while as you share food, conversation, or whatever activities bring your chosen family together.

RITUAL FOR LIFE TRANSITIONS AND MILESTONES

LGBTQ+ lives include unique milestones and transitions that mainstream culture often doesn't recognize.

Creating rituals around these moments helps honor their significance and strengthens community support.

The Coming Out Celebration

When someone in your community comes out or reaches a new level of openness about their identity:

What you need: A gift that represents their identity (rainbow item, book by LGBTQ+ authors, etc.), flowers, and community members who want to celebrate

Present the gift and say: "We celebrate your courage in living your truth. We honor the journey that brought you to this moment of authenticity. We welcome you more fully into our community and commit to supporting you as you continue to grow."

Have each community member share one thing they appreciate about the person or one way they're excited to support them going forward.

The Name Change Ceremony

When someone legally or socially changes their name:

What you need: Something to write with, paper, and a way to safely burn paper

Have the person write their old name on one piece of paper and their new name on another. The community gathers in a circle around them.

Say together: "We witness this transformation. We release the name that no longer serves and welcome the name that honors your truth."

The person burns the old name paper (safely) and keeps the new name paper. Everyone practices saying the new name with love and intention.

The Transition Milestone Blessing

For any significant transition milestone (starting hormones, surgery, legal gender marker changes, etc.):
What you need: Blue candles for healing, a photo of the person, and small gifts from community members
Light the blue candles and place the photo in the center. Each community member places a small gift (this can be as simple as a written note) near the photo while sharing a blessing or wish for the person's continued journey.
End with: "We bless this step in your journey toward wholeness. We celebrate your courage and commitment to authentic living. We hold you in love through all your transformations."

GRIEF AND MEMORIAL MAGIC

Queer life includes joy, but also loss — of relationships, of family acceptance, of community members to violence, illness, or neglect. Magic can help us honor grief without being consumed by it.

Our community has experienced profound losses – from the AIDS epidemic to suicide, violence, and other tragedies. Creating space for collective grief and healing is crucial for community wellbeing.

Candle of Mourning

Light a black or white candle. Speak the name(s) of who or what you've lost. Say:
"I honor this grief. I honor this love. I carry memory forward, and I release the weight."

River Release Ritual

Write what you're grieving on a piece of paper. Tear it

into strips and release them into running water (stream, sink, even shower). Visualize the grief flowing away, leaving space for healing.

Resilience Charm

Carry a stone or coin and whisper to it:
"I have survived before. I will survive again."
Keep it with you as a touchstone when things feel overwhelming.

The Community Grief Ritual

For processing collective grief (after community losses, during Transgender Day of Remembrance, etc.):
What you need: Black candles for releasing grief, white candles for honoring those who've passed, tissues, and a safe space for emotions

Light the black candles and invite people to share their grief, anger, or sadness. Don't try to fix or minimize these feelings – just hold space for them.

After people have shared, light the white candles and invite people to share memories of those they're grieving or qualities they want to honor.

End by saying together: "We carry our grief because we carry love. We honor those we've lost by living fully, loving boldly, and caring for each other."

The Memorial Altar

Create a community space that honors LGBTQ+ folks who've passed away:
What you need: Photos, names, or symbols representing those you want to honor, flowers, and candles

This might be a temporary altar for a specific memorial service, or a permanent space in a community center.

Include:

- Photos of community members who've passed
- Names of LGBTQ+ folks lost to violence or suicide
- Symbols representing broader losses (like a ribbon for AIDS victims)

Keep fresh flowers and lit candles when possible. Encourage community members to visit, leave offerings, and share memories.

The Healing Circle Practice

For ongoing community healing from trauma and loss:
What you need: A regular group of people committed to showing up for each other
Meet regularly (monthly or quarterly) to:

- Check in on how people are processing grief and trauma
- Share resources for healing and support
- Practice healing activities together (meditation, breathwork, creative expression)
- Plan ways to support community members who are struggling

Open each gathering by acknowledging that healing is ongoing and that you're committed to supporting each other through the process.

ACTIVISM AND SOCIAL JUSTICE MAGIC

Many LGBTQ+ folks are called to activism and social justice work. Magic can support these efforts and help sustain activists through challenging times.

The Activist Protection Spell

Before protests, activism events, or other potentially challenging social justice work:
What you need: A piece of black tourmaline or another protective stone, and clear intention
Hold the stone and charge it with protective energy. Set the intention that it will:

- Keep you physically and emotionally safe during activism work
- Help you stay grounded and focused on your goals
- Protect you from absorbing others' anger or negativity
- Give you strength to continue fighting for justice

Carry this stone during activism activities and hold it when you need extra strength or protection.

The Justice Manifestation Ritual

For supporting longer-term social justice goals:
What you need: Purple candles (for justice), a map of your area, and clear intentions about what changes you want to see
Light the purple candles and place them around the map. Visualize the specific changes you want to see in your community – marriage equality, employment protections, inclusive healthcare, safe schools, etc.
Say: "We call forth justice and equality for all LGBTQ+ people. We manifest a world where everyone can live authentically and safely. Our activism is supported by the universe itself."
Focus your energy on both the ideal future you want to create and the concrete steps needed to get there.

The Activist Burnout Prevention Practice

Activism can be emotionally and physically draining. This practice helps maintain sustainable energy for long-term social justice work:

What you need: Green candles for renewal, a bowl of water, and mint or another refreshing herb

Light the green candles and add mint to the water. Dip your fingers in the mint water and touch your heart, saying:

"I renew my commitment to justice while honoring my own needs for rest and restoration. I sustain my activism through self-care and community support. I am part of a movement larger than myself."

Use this practice regularly to prevent burnout and maintain perspective on your role in larger social change efforts.

Online Community Magic

Many LGBTQ+ folks connect primarily through online communities, especially those in rural areas or who haven't found local community yet. These practices help strengthen virtual connections and create sacred space online.

The Digital Sacred Space Blessing

Before joining online LGBTQ+ groups or communities:

What you need: Your computer or phone, and clear intentions about how you want to show up online

Place your hands on your device and say: "I bless this technology that connects me with my community. I commit to showing up authentically and supportively in online spaces. I attract meaningful connections and avoid toxic interactions."

Set intentions about how you want to engage online – sharing authentically, supporting others, avoiding drama, etc.

The Virtual Gathering Blessing

For online LGBTQ+ events, support groups, or social gatherings:
What you need: Participants willing to do a brief opening ritual
Begin the gathering by having everyone light a candle on their end (or hold their hand to their heart if candles aren't possible). Say together:
"Though we're physically separated, we gather in spirit. We create sacred space through our shared intention to support and celebrate each other. Our online community is real and powerful."
This helps create a sense of connection and intention even when people are joining from different locations.

The Digital Detox Ritual

Online spaces can sometimes become overwhelming or toxic. This ritual helps you cleanse from negative online interactions:
What you need: A bowl of salt water, a soft cloth, and your electronic devices
Dip the cloth in salt water and gently wipe down your devices (being careful not to damage them). As you do this, say:
"I cleanse these tools of any negative energy they've absorbed. I release toxic interactions and focus on positive connections. I engage online in ways that support my wellbeing."

FAMILY HOLIDAY MAGIC

Many LGBTQ+ folks face challenges during family holidays – whether from lack of acceptance, complicated family dynamics, or simply feeling different from relatives. These practices help you navigate family time while staying true to yourself.

The Family Holiday Protection Spell

Before family gatherings that might be challenging:
What you need: A small object you can keep in your pocket, and protective intentions

Charge the object with protective energy by visualizing it surrounded by white light. Set the intention that it will:

- Help you stay centered in your own truth
- Give you strength to maintain appropriate boundaries
- Protect you from absorbing family drama or negativity
- Remind you that you have chosen family who loves you unconditionally

Touch this object whenever you need to reconnect with your strength during family events.

The Chosen Family Holiday Ritual

Create your own holiday celebrations with chosen family:
What you need: Your chosen family members and whatever traditions feel meaningful to you

This might include:

- Sharing what you're grateful for about your chosen family
- Exchanging gifts that honor each person's authentic identity
- Creating new traditions that celebrate your community
- Blessing the food and the gathering with intentions of love and acceptance

Say together: "We create our own traditions rooted in authentic love and acceptance. Our chosen family celebrations are sacred and meaningful."

The Holiday Gratitude Practice

Focus on what you're genuinely grateful for during challenging holiday seasons:

Each day during holiday seasons, write down three things you're grateful for related to your LGBTQ+ identity or community. These might include:

- Friends who accept you completely
- Progress you've made in self-acceptance
- LGBTQ+ activists who've created more opportunities
- Online communities that provide support
- Small moments of authentic connection

This practice helps shift focus from what's difficult to what's genuinely positive in your life.

Making Community Magic Sustainable

The most effective community magic becomes part of regular life rather than something you only do during special events.

Here are ways to maintain magical community connections:

Regular community appreciation practices where you send loving energy to LGBTQ+ folks in your area

Monthly chosen family check-ins to maintain close relationships

Seasonal community service that serves LGBTQ+ causes you care about

Online community engagement that's positive and supportive

Mentoring younger LGBTQ+ folks and learning from elders

Creating inclusive spaces wherever you have influence

The Ripple Effect

Remember that your community magic creates ripple effects far beyond what you can see. Every time you create inclusive space, every time you show up authentically in community, every time you support another LGBTQ+ person's journey, you're contributing to a larger transformation.

Your magic helps create the kind of world where all LGBTQ+ people can thrive. It builds communities where young people can see positive examples of queer adulthood, where elders are honored and supported, where everyone's authentic self is celebrated.

This is some of the most important magic you can do – the magic of building beloved community where everyone belongs.

CHAPTER 7
Everyday Magic for Extraordinary Lives

The most powerful magic often happens in the small, daily moments – the morning ritual that sets your intention for the day, the commute visualization that helps you arrive centered and confident, the bedtime practice that processes the day's experiences and prepares you for restful sleep.

This chapter is about integrating magic seamlessly into your everyday life as an LGBTQ+ person. These aren't elaborate rituals that require hours of preparation – they're simple, practical magical practices that fit into busy schedules and real-world constraints while helping you navigate the unique challenges and celebrate the unique joys of queer life.

Morning Magic: Starting Your Day with Intention

How you begin your day sets the energetic tone for everything that follows. These morning practices help you center yourself in your authentic identity and prepare for whatever the day might bring.

The Authentic Self Check-In

Before you even get out of bed, place your hand on your heart and ask yourself: "Who am I today, and how do I want to show up in the world?"

This isn't about creating a fake persona – it's about consciously connecting with your authentic self and setting an intention for how you want to embody that authenticity throughout the day.

Your answer might be:

- "I am confident and creative, and I want to share my ideas boldly"
- "I am compassionate and strong, and I want to support others while honoring my own boundaries"
- "I am curious and open, and I want to learn something new about myself or the world"
- "I am resilient and joyful, and I want to find moments of celebration even in ordinary experiences"

The Mirror Affirmation Practice

While getting ready in the morning, make eye contact with yourself in the mirror and say one genuinely positive thing about yourself. This can be about your appearance, your character, your growth, or anything you honestly appreciate.

If mirror work feels challenging, start small:

- "I see someone who's brave enough to live authentically"
- "I appreciate how hard I'm working to grow and change"
- "I'm grateful for my unique perspective on the world"
- "I see someone worthy of love and respect"

The key is authenticity – say things you can genuinely believe, even if they feel unfamiliar at first.

The Daily Shield Visualization

As part of your morning routine (while brushing teeth, making coffee, or commuting), visualize yourself surrounded by protective, confident energy.

This shield is permeable – it lets love, opportunities, and positive energy flow freely in and out, but it deflects judgment, discrimination, and other people's negative emotions.

Set the intention: "I move through today protected and confident. I attract positive interactions and opportunities. I stay centered in my own truth regardless of external circumstances."

The Gratitude Foundation

Before leaving home each morning, identify three things you're genuinely grateful for. At least one should be related to your LGBTQ+ identity or community.

This might include:

- Friends who use your correct pronouns automatically
- Progress you've made in self-acceptance
- The freedom to express your authentic style
- Online communities that provide support and connection
- Legal protections that previous generations fought for

This practice trains your brain to notice positive aspects of your queer experience, which makes it easier to maintain perspective during challenging moments.

COMMUTE AND TRANSPORTATION MAGIC

Whether you're walking, driving, or using public transportation, travel time offers opportunities for magical practice that can transform your arrival energy at work, social events, or anywhere else you're going.

The Journey Blessing

At the beginning of any trip, take a moment to bless your journey:

"I travel safely and arrive exactly when I'm meant to. My journey is smooth and peaceful. I attract helpful, friendly people along the way."

This works for everything from daily commutes to major trips, and it helps you approach travel with calm confidence rather than anxiety.

The Destination Visualization

During your commute, spend time visualizing yourself arriving at your destination feeling confident, prepared, and authentically yourself.

If you're heading to work, see yourself walking in with good posture, greeting colleagues warmly, and handling whatever challenges arise with competence and grace.

If you're going to a social event, visualize yourself enjoying genuine connections, feeling comfortable in your own skin, and contributing positively to whatever gathering you're attending.

This mental rehearsal helps you actually embody these qualities when you arrive.

The Traffic Light Meditation

When you're stopped at red lights (or waiting for public transportation), use the time for brief centering practices:

Take three deep breaths and remind yourself: "I am exactly where I need to be. I trust the timing of my day. I approach each moment with patience and presence."

This transforms frustrating delays into opportunities for mindfulness and stress reduction.

The Public Transportation Shield

If you use public transportation and sometimes feel vulnerable or uncomfortable:

Visualize yourself surrounded by a bubble of protective light that makes you essentially invisible to anyone who might want to cause trouble, while making you easily visible to helpful, friendly people.

Set the intention: "I travel safely and comfortably. I attract respectful interactions and avoid conflicts. I arrive at my destination feeling calm and centered."

WORKPLACE MAGIC THROUGHOUT THE DAY

Work environments can present ongoing challenges for LGBTQ+ folks – from microaggressions to decisions about disclosure to general workplace stress. These practices help you maintain your authentic self while navigating professional demands.

The Monday Morning Reset

At the beginning of each work week, take a few minutes to set magical intentions for the week ahead:

"I approach this week with confidence and competence. I contribute my unique perspective and skills. I maintain professional relationships while staying true to myself. I attract opportunities for growth and recognition."

The Email/Message Blessing

Before opening your email or messages each day, especially if you're expecting potentially stressful communications:

Place your hands on your computer or phone and visualize white light flowing into your inbox, neutralizing any negative energy and highlighting messages that require your attention while allowing less important items to wait.

Set the intention: "I receive only communications that serve my highest good today. I respond to everything with clarity and professionalism. I maintain appropriate boundaries around my time and energy."

The Difficult Conversation Preparation

Before challenging work conversations (performance reviews, coming out to colleagues, addressing discrimination, etc.):

Take several deep breaths and visualize the conversation going well. See yourself speaking clearly and confidently, the other person listening respectfully, and both of you reaching positive outcomes.

Hold a small confidence charm (stone, jewelry, or even a coin) and set the intention: "I speak my truth with courage and clarity. I am heard and respected. This conversation serves the highest good of everyone involved."

The Lunch Break Restoration

Use part of your lunch break for magical restoration rather than just eating:

Find a quiet space (even if it's just your car or a bathroom stall) and do a quick energy cleansing. Visualize any workplace stress, frustration, or negative energy flowing out of your body and being replaced with calm, confident energy.

Say: "I release the morning's stress and begin the afternoon refreshed. I return to work centered and capable. I maintain my energy and enthusiasm throughout the day."

The End-of-Workday Transition

Before leaving work each day, perform a brief ritual to transition from professional to personal energy:

Visualize removing an invisible work uniform and putting on clothes that represent your authentic self (even if your actual clothes don't change).

Say: "I appreciate the work I accomplished today. I leave work stress at work and return to my personal life with energy and joy. I am free to be fully myself."

This helps prevent work stress from contaminating your personal time and relationships.

SOCIAL SITUATION MAGIC

Social interactions can be complex for LGBTQ+ folks – whether we're navigating mixed groups where not everyone is affirming, deciding how much of ourselves to reveal, or simply dealing with social anxiety that might be heightened by identity concerns.

The Party Preparation Ritual

Before social events where you're not sure how accepting the environment will be:

Choose your outfit with intention, picking clothing that makes you feel confident and authentic. As you get dressed, visualize each piece of clothing as armor that protects your authentic self while allowing genuine connections to form.

Say: "I go to this gathering as my authentic self. I attract people who appreciate and respect who I am. I enjoy genuine connections and gracefully avoid anyone who doesn't serve my highest good."

The Small Talk Blessing

For situations where you need to engage in small talk but want to stay authentic:

Before the interaction, set the intention: "I engage authentically within appropriate boundaries. I find common ground with others while honoring my own truth. I contribute positively to conversations without compromising my integrity."

This helps you be friendly and professional without feeling like you're hiding or pretending to be someone you're not.

The Coming Out Moment Support

When you decide to come out to someone in the moment:

Take a deep breath and quickly visualize yourself surrounded by the love of everyone who already accepts you. Feel their support strengthening you.

Say silently: "I speak my truth with courage. I deserve to be known and accepted for who I am. However this person responds, I remain whole and valuable."

The Social Energy Management

During long social events, especially those that require emotional labor or vigilance:

Periodically step away (to the bathroom, outside for air, etc.) and do a quick energy reset. Visualize any heavy or draining energy flowing out of your body and being replaced with light, positive energy.

Touch your heart and remind yourself: "I maintain my energy and boundaries. I engage authentically without depleting myself. I honor both my need for connection and my need for self-care."

DATING AND RELATIONSHIP MAGIC

Romantic relationships require ongoing magical attention – not to manipulate outcomes, but to help you stay centered, authentic, and open to genuine connection.

The Dating App Daily Blessing

Each time you open dating apps:
Hold your phone and set the intention: "I attract people who are genuinely interested in getting to know the real me. I recognize good matches easily and avoid wasting time on incompatible people. I approach dating with curiosity and joy rather than desperation or fear."

The Pre-Date Centering

Before any date, whether first dates or regular time with a long-term partner:
Take a few minutes to connect with yourself and your intentions for the interaction. Say: "I show up as my authentic self. I am curious about this person while maintaining my own boundaries and standards. I enjoy this time regardless of the ultimate outcome."

The Relationship Check-In Magic

For people in relationships, do a weekly magical check-in:

Light a candle and ask yourself: "How am I showing up in this relationship? What does my partner need from me? What do I need from them? How can we both grow while staying connected?"

Don't try to magically change your partner – focus on your own growth and contribution to the relationship's health.

The Breakup Processing Ritual

When relationships end, use magic to process emotions and move forward healthily:

Write everything you're feeling on paper – sadness, anger, gratitude, relief, whatever comes up. Burn the paper safely while saying: "I honor all my feelings about this relationship. I keep the lessons and release the pain. I am open to love again when the time is right."

DIGITAL LIFE MAGIC

Since so much of modern life happens online, it makes sense to bring magical awareness to our digital interactions.

The Social Media Blessing

Before opening social media apps:

Set the intention: "I see content that uplifts and informs me. I engage in ways that spread positivity and connection. I avoid toxic interactions and remember that online personas aren't complete pictures of people's lives."

The Digital Cleansing Practice

Weekly, do a magical cleansing of your digital devices:
Hold your phone, computer, or tablet and visualize white light flowing through them, clearing out any negative energy they've absorbed from toxic online interactions, stressful work communications, or overwhelming news consumption.

Say: "I cleanse these tools of negative energy. They serve my highest good and connect me with positive information and relationships."

The Online Dating Profile Blessing

When creating or updating dating profiles:
Before posting photos or writing descriptions, hold your hands over your device and say: "This profile attracts people who will appreciate my authentic self. It repels those who wouldn't be good matches. It presents me honestly and appealingly."

The News and Media Boundaries

Before consuming news or social media content:
Set clear intentions about how much time you'll spend and what kind of content serves your wellbeing. Say: "I stay informed about things I care about without becoming overwhelmed. I balance awareness with self-care. I engage with media in ways that empower rather than drain me."

EVENING AND BEDTIME MAGIC

How you end your day is just as important as how you begin it. Evening practices help you process the day's experiences, release stress, and prepare for restorative sleep.

The Daily Gratitude and Release

Each evening, mentally review your day and identify:
- Three things you're genuinely grateful for
- One thing you're proud of accomplishing (however small)
- One thing you're ready to release or let go of

This practice helps you end each day with appreciation while preventing stress from accumulating.

The Authenticity Appreciation

Before bed, think of one moment during the day when you felt genuinely authentic – when you expressed yourself honestly, made a choice that honored your values, or simply felt comfortable in your own skin.

Appreciate that moment and say: "I celebrate my commitment to authentic living. Each day I become more myself. I am grateful for my courage in being real in a world that often rewards pretense."

The Tomorrow Intention Setting

As you're falling asleep, set a gentle intention for the following day: "Tomorrow I approach each situation with confidence and authenticity. I attract positive interactions and opportunities. I handle challenges with grace and maintain connection to my true self throughout the day."

This plants seeds in your subconscious mind that can influence how you show up the next day.

The Worry Transformation Practice

If you're lying awake worrying about tomorrow's challenges:

Visualize each worry as a bubble floating away from you. As it floats away, it transforms from a problem into a possibility – a chance to practice your strengths, learn something new, or connect more deeply with your authentic self.

Say: "I release today's worries and tomorrow's unknowns. I trust my ability to handle whatever comes. I sleep peacefully knowing I am exactly who I'm meant to be."

SEASONAL MAGIC FOR LGBTQ+ LIVES

Each season offers unique opportunities for magical practice that honors both natural cycles and the specific rhythms of queer life.

Spring: New Growth and Fresh Starts

Use spring energy for:

- Setting intentions for personal growth and self-discovery
- Blessing new relationships or deepening existing ones
- Starting creative projects that express your authentic self
- Cleaning out belongings that no longer reflect who you're becoming

Summer: Visibility and Celebration

Use summer energy for:

- Celebrating Pride and your identity

- Taking risks that help you grow and expand
- Building community connections and chosen family bonds
- Expressing yourself boldly and joyfully

Fall: Harvest and Gratitude

Use fall energy for:

- Appreciating how far you've come in your personal journey
- Honoring the support you've received from community
- Preparing for challenging seasons with self-care practices
- Releasing relationships or situations that no longer serve you

Winter: Rest and Reflection

Use winter energy for:

- Deep self-reflection about your growth and goals
- Cozy gatherings with chosen family
- Planning for the year ahead
- Honoring your need for rest and restoration

EMERGENCY MAGIC FOR DIFFICULT DAYS

Some days are harder than others – whether due to discrimination, rejection, health challenges, or simply the accumulated stress of living authentically in a sometimes hostile world. These practices provide quick magical support during difficult times.

The Instant Confidence Boost

When you need immediate confidence support:
Place your hand on your heart and take three deep breaths. Say: "I am worthy of respect and love. I have every right to exist authentically. I am stronger than any challenge I face."

Visualize golden light filling your chest and radiating outward, reminding you of your inherent worth and power.

The Support Network Visualization

When you're feeling alone or overwhelmed:
Close your eyes and visualize yourself surrounded by everyone who truly loves and supports you – friends, chosen family, supportive relatives, mentors, even pets. Feel their love surrounding you like a warm embrace.

Say: "I am never truly alone. I am held in a network of love and support. I can ask for help when I need it."

The "This Too Shall Pass" Ritual

During particularly difficult experiences:
Hold a small object (stone, coin, piece of jewelry) and visualize all your current pain, stress, or fear flowing into it. Say: "This difficulty is temporary. I have survived hard times before and will survive this too. I am resilient and capable of healing."

Keep the object for a day or two as a reminder that painful feelings are temporary, then release it (throw it in a river, bury it, or simply throw it away) as a symbol of releasing the pain.

Making Everyday Magic Sustainable

The key to effective everyday magic is consistency rather

than perfection. You don't need to do every practice every day – choose the ones that resonate with you and adapt them to fit your life.

Start small with one or two practices that feel manageable

Be flexible and modify practices to fit your schedule and circumstances

Focus on intention rather than perfect execution

Track what works by paying attention to which practices actually improve your daily experience

Build gradually by adding new practices only after existing ones feel natural

Be compassionate with yourself when you forget or skip practices

The Ripple Effects of Daily Magic

Remember that your everyday magic doesn't just benefit you – it influences everyone around you. When you start your day centered and confident, that energy affects every interaction you have. When you move through the world with authentic self-love, you give others permission to do the same.

Your daily magical practices contribute to a more magical world for all LGBTQ+ people. Every time you choose authenticity over conformity, every time you respond to challenges with grace instead of reactivity, every time you treat yourself with the love and respect you deserve, you're modeling possibilities for others.

The ordinary moments of your extraordinary queer life are opportunities for magic. The commute where you practice self-affirmation, the difficult conversation where you stay centered in your truth, the evening when you appreciate your own growth – these moments matter more than you might realize.

Your life is already magical. These practices just help you notice and amplify the magic that's already there.

CHAPTER 8
Building Your Long-Term Practice

Magic isn't a quick fix or a one-time solution – it's a practice that grows and evolves with you throughout your life. As an LGBTQ+ person, your magical practice can provide stability and grounding as you navigate the ongoing process of becoming more authentically yourself, building community, and creating the kind of life you truly want.

This chapter is about sustaining your magical practice over time, adapting it as you grow and change, and integrating it so deeply into your life that it becomes as natural as breathing. We'll also address what to do when spells don't seem to work, how to deepen your knowledge, and ways to connect with other magical practitioners in the LGBTQ+ community.

CREATING SUSTAINABLE MAGICAL HABITS

The most powerful magic happens through consistent, small actions rather than elaborate occasional rituals. Building sustainable habits means finding practices that fit your actual life, not some idealized version of it.

The Five-Minute Daily Practice

Choose one simple magical practice you can commit to

doing every day for five minutes or less. This might be:

- Morning affirmations while getting ready
- Brief gratitude practice before bed
- Protective visualization during your commute
- Self-love check-in while brushing teeth
- Intention setting while making coffee

The key is choosing something so simple that you can do it even on your worst days. Once this becomes automatic (usually 3-4 weeks), you can add additional practices if you want to.

The Weekly Magical Check-In

Every week, spend 10-15 minutes reviewing your magical practice:

- What's working well for you right now?
- What feels forced or inauthentic?
- What challenges are you facing that might benefit from magical support?
- How has your practice supported your growth and goals?
- What adjustments do you want to make for the coming week?

This prevents your practice from becoming stale or disconnected from your actual needs.

The Monthly Practice Evolution

Once a month, take a longer look at your magical practice:

- How has your practice changed over the past month?
- What new techniques do you want to try?
- What aspects of your identity or life need more magical attention?
- How can you deepen the practices that are serving you well?
- What resources or learning opportunities interest you?

Allow your practice to grow and change as you do. What worked perfectly six months ago might not fit your current life or goals.

SEASONAL PRACTICE ADJUSTMENTS

Adapt your magical practice to match the seasons and the natural rhythms of LGBTQ+ community life:

Winter (January-March):

Focus on introspection, planning, and building inner strength for the year ahead. This is a good time for deep self-reflection, goal setting, and practices that support mental and emotional health during potentially challenging months.

Spring (April-June):

Emphasize growth, new beginnings, and preparation for Pride season. Focus on practices that support visibility, confidence, and community building as you prepare for increased social activity.

Summer (July-September):

Center celebration, community, and visibility. This is Pride season and the time for practices that support bold self-expression, community engagement, and managing the intensity of increased social and political activity.

Fall (October-December):

Focus on gratitude, harvest, and preparation for winter. This is a good time for practices that honor your growth, strengthen relationships, and prepare for holiday seasons that might involve challenging family dynamics.

WHEN SPELLS DON'T WORK (& WHY THAT'S OKAY)

Every magical practitioner experiences times when spells don't seem to produce the desired results. This is normal and doesn't mean you're doing anything wrong or that magic doesn't work. Understanding why spells sometimes don't work can actually deepen your practice and make you more effective over time.

COMMON REASONS SPELLS MAY NOT WORK AS EXPECTED

Conflicted intentions:

If part of you wants something but another part is afraid of it, your magical energy gets scattered. For example, you might do a spell to attract a romantic partner while simultaneously believing you don't deserve love.

Unrealistic timelines:

Magic works with natural timing, which isn't always the

same as our preferred timing. A spell for career change might take months to manifest as you build skills, make connections, and find the right opportunities.

Focusing on outcomes instead of growth:

Spells that try to control specific people or force particular outcomes often backfire. Magic works better when it focuses on your own growth, confidence, and ability to recognize and seize opportunities.

Lack of follow-through:

Magic without action rarely produces results. If you do a spell for a new job but don't update your resume or apply for positions, you're not giving the magic practical channels to work through.

Mismatched energy:

Sometimes what we think we want isn't what we actually need or what would truly make us happy. Magic has a way of redirecting us toward what serves our highest good, even if it's different from our original request.

WHAT TO DO WHEN SPELLS DON'T WORK

Examine your true desires:

Ask yourself honestly whether you really want what you asked for, or whether there might be something deeper driving your request.

Look for partial results:

Magic often works in unexpected ways. You might not

have gotten exactly what you asked for, but have you experienced any positive changes related to your spell?

Consider divine timing:

Some things need to happen at specific times or in specific sequences. Trust that delays might be protecting you or preparing you for something better.

Take practical action:

Make sure you're giving your magic concrete ways to work. Combine spells with practical steps toward your goals.

Try different approaches:

If one type of spell isn't working, experiment with different techniques. Some people respond better to visualization, others to candle magic, others to written spells.

Check for blocks:

Are there beliefs, fears, or past experiences that might be interfering with your magical work? Sometimes we need healing or clearing work before manifestation spells can be effective.

When to Let Go

Sometimes the most magical thing you can do is release attachment to a specific outcome and trust that the universe has something better in store. Signs it might be time to let go include:

- You've tried multiple approaches over several months with no movement
- Pursuing this goal is causing significant stress or unhappiness
- You're starting to realize this goal doesn't actually align with your values or authentic self
- Unexpected opportunities are arising that interest you more than your original goal

Remember: letting go isn't giving up. It's trusting that your magical practice has opened you to possibilities you might not have considered before.

DEEPENING YOUR KNOWLEDGE

As you become more comfortable with basic magical practices, you might want to expand your knowledge and skills. Here are ways to deepen your understanding while staying true to your LGBTQ+ identity and values.

Reading and Research

Start with LGBTQ+-affirming authors who understand the intersection of queerness and spirituality. Look for books that honor diverse spiritual traditions without requiring you to fit into rigid categories.

Explore different magical traditions that appeal to you – witchcraft, chaos magic, folk magic, ceremonial magic, or others. Take what resonates and leave what doesn't.

Study the history of LGBTQ+ people in magical and spiritual traditions. Understanding our ancestral connections to these practices can deepen your sense of belonging.

Learn about herbalism, astrology, tarot, or other specialties that interest you. Each adds new dimensions to your magical toolkit.

Critical thinking approach: Always read magical material with discernment. Just because something is published doesn't mean it's accurate or appropriate for your path.

Experimentation and Practice

Keep a magical journal where you record spells, their results, observations about your practice, and insights about what works for you.

Try new techniques regularly, but give each one enough time to see if it fits your natural style and produces results.

Seasonal experiments: Use the changing seasons as opportunities to explore different types of magic – purification in spring, abundance in summer, gratitude in fall, introspection in winter.

Collaborate with others who share your interest in both magic and LGBTQ+ identity. Teaching and learning from community deepens everyone's practice.

Mentorship and Teaching

Seek mentors who understand both magical practice and LGBTQ+ experience. This might be through formal spiritual communities, online groups, or informal relationships with more experienced practitioners.

Teach others as you learn. Sharing your knowledge with newer practitioners helps solidify your own understanding and contributes to LGBTQ+ magical community.

Cross-pollination: Learn from practitioners of different backgrounds while maintaining your own authentic approach.

Connecting with LGBTQ+ Magical Community

Magic can be deeply personal, but it's often enhanced by community connection. Finding other LGBTQ+ folks who share your interest in magical practice can provide support, inspiration, and opportunities for group work.

Online Communities

Social media groups focused on queer spirituality, LGBTQ+ witchcraft, or similar topics can provide daily connection and support.

Video calls and virtual gatherings allow you to participate in group rituals and discussions even if you don't have local community.

Online learning opportunities like webinars, courses, or workshops specifically designed for LGBTQ+ practitioners.

Forum discussions where you can ask questions, share experiences, and learn from others' approaches to magical practice.

Local Community Building

LGBTQ+ centers sometimes host spiritual or metaphysical discussion groups, even if they're not explicitly magical.

Pagan or metaphysical shops in LGBTQ+-friendly areas often have bulletin boards or know about local groups.

University LGBTQ+ groups sometimes include members interested in alternative spirituality and magical practice.

Create your own group by starting small with friends who share your interests, then growing through word of mouth.

Pride and community events often attract people with

diverse spiritual interests who might be open to magical community.

Group Practice Considerations

When participating in group magical work, consider:

Consent and boundaries: Make sure everyone is comfortable with the types of magic being practiced and has the right to opt out of anything that doesn't feel right.

Inclusive language: Use language that honors everyone's gender identity, relationship structure, and spiritual background.

Shared values: While you don't all need identical beliefs, successful magical groups usually share core values about things like consent, harm reduction, and mutual respect.

Leadership structure: Decide whether you want rotating leadership, collective decision-making, or more formal hierarchy.

Practical considerations: Meeting location, timing, supplies, and costs should be accessible to all members.

Integrating Magic with Other Life Areas

A mature magical practice doesn't exist in isolation – it integrates seamlessly with your career, relationships, activism, creativity, and other important life areas.

Magic and Professional Life

Ethical considerations: Consider how your magical practice informs your professional ethics and decision-making without imposing your beliefs on others.

Workplace applications: Use magical practices for confidence, clarity, and stress management without necessarily discussing your spiritual path with colleagues.

Career guidance: Let your magical practice help you

discern which career paths truly align with your authentic self and values.

Leadership development: As you advance professionally, use magical principles like energy management and intuition to become a more effective leader.

Magic and Relationships

Healthy boundaries: Use magical practice to maintain appropriate boundaries in all relationships – romantic, family, friendship, and professional.

Authentic communication: Let magic help you communicate more honestly and effectively, especially about difficult topics.

Conflict resolution: Apply magical principles like grounding and centering to navigate relationship challenges with greater skill.

Community building: Use your magical practice to contribute to building stronger, more supportive LGBTQ+ community.

Magic and Activism

Sustainable engagement: Use magical practices to maintain energy and hope for long-term activism without burning out.

Strategic thinking: Let magical practice help you discern which causes and activities deserve your limited time and energy.

Emotional regulation: Apply magical techniques to manage anger, frustration, and grief related to social justice work.

Visionary planning: Use magical practice to maintain

focus on the world you want to create, not just the problems you want to solve.

Magic and Creativity

Inspiration: Use magical practice to access creative inspiration and overcome blocks.

Authentic expression: Let magic help you express your unique perspective and experiences through creative work.

Professional development: Apply magical principles to building creative careers that honor both your artistic vision and practical needs.

Community contribution: Use creative work as a form of magical practice that contributes to LGBTQ+ visibility and community building.

Advanced Practices for Long-Term Practitioners

As your practice matures, you might want to explore more complex or specialized forms of magic that build on the foundation you've established.

Seasonal and Lunar Cycles

Moon phase magic: Align your magical work with lunar cycles – new moons for new beginnings, full moons for manifestation and celebration, waning moons for release and healing.

Seasonal celebrations: Create or adapt traditional seasonal celebrations to honor both natural cycles and LGBTQ+ community milestones.

Personal cycles: Pay attention to your own energy cycles and plan magical work accordingly – some people are more magically effective at certain times of day, month, or year.

Divination and Intuition Development

Tarot, oracle cards, or other divination systems can provide guidance for magical work and life decisions.

Meditation and mindfulness practices deepen your connection to intuition and inner wisdom.

Dream work can provide insights and guidance for both magical practice and daily life.

Energy sensing and reading helps you better understand the energetic effects of your magical work.

Advanced Spellwork

Layered spells that work on multiple levels – mental, emotional, spiritual, and practical.

Long-term manifestation projects that unfold over months or years rather than days or weeks.

Group ritual leadership where you facilitate magical work for community rather than just personal practice.

Healing work that addresses trauma, family-of-origin issues, or internalized oppression through magical means.

Dealing with Spiritual Bypassing and Toxic Positivity

As your magical practice deepens, it's important to avoid using spirituality to avoid dealing with real problems or uncomfortable emotions. This is especially important for LGBTQ+ folks who may face genuine discrimination and systemic challenges.

Recognizing Spiritual Bypassing

Using magic as a substitute for practical action, therapy, or medical care when those are what's actually needed.

Dismissing legitimate anger about discrimination or injustice as "negative energy" that should be avoided.

Believing that positive thinking alone can overcome systemic oppression or serious mental health issues.

Avoiding difficult emotions by trying to maintain constant positivity or spiritual "high vibes."

Blaming yourself for negative experiences, believing they're all the result of your thoughts or energy.

Maintaining Balance

Magic plus action: Use magical practice to support practical efforts rather than replace them.

Emotional honesty: Allow yourself to feel the full range of human emotions, including anger, sadness, and fear, while using magical practice to process them healthily.

Systemic awareness: Recognize that some problems are systemic rather than personal and require collective action, not just individual magical work.

Professional help: Use therapy, medical care, and other professional resources alongside magical practice when appropriate.

Community support: Balance individual magical practice with involvement in LGBTQ+ community and social justice work.

Your Magic, Your Path

As you develop a long-term magical practice, remember that your path is unique. What works for other practitioners might not work for you, and that's perfectly fine. The goal isn't to become like other magical practitioners – it's to become more authentically yourself.

Your queerness is an asset in magical practice, not something to overcome or work around. Your lived experience of transformation, authenticity, and resilience gives you natural magical abilities that many people spend years trying to develop. Your perspective as an LGBTQ+ person brings unique insights and approaches to magical work.

Trust your instincts about what practices serve you and what don't. Adapt techniques to fit your life, beliefs, and goals. Create new practices when existing ones don't quite meet your needs. Share your innovations with community when appropriate.

Most importantly, let your magical practice support you in becoming the person you're meant to be. Let it help you love yourself more fully, build stronger community connections, navigate challenges with greater grace, and contribute to creating a more magical world for all LGBTQ+ people.

Your practice is a gift – to yourself, to your community, and to the world. Honor it, nurture it, and let it grow with you throughout your life.

APPENDIX

SUPPLIES AND TOOLS

Basic Magical Supplies (Budget-Friendly Options):

- Candles: Any color, any size - even birthday candles work for spells
- Salt: Regular table salt for cleansing and protection
- Herbs: Start with kitchen herbs like rosemary, thyme, and cinnamon
- Stones: Clear quartz and black tourmaline are versatile starter stones
- Incense: Sage, cedar, or any scent that feels cleansing to you
- Journal: Any notebook for recording spells and experiences

Where to Shop:

- Local metaphysical shops (support small businesses when possible)
- Health food stores (for herbs and natural supplies)
- Craft stores (for candles, bowls, and other tools)
- Online retailers (for harder-to-find items)
- Nature walks (for stones, leaves, and other natural materials)

LGBTQ+-Owned Magical Businesses:

- Research local LGBTQ+-owned metaphysical shops in your area
- Look for online shops run by queer practitioners
- Support LGBTQ+ authors by buying books directly from them when possible

- Attend Pride events that include pagan or spiritual vendors

BUILDING YOUR MAGICAL LIBRARY

Start with these types of books:

- One general witchcraft/magic book that resonates with you
- One book specifically about LGBTQ+ spirituality or experience
- One book about a specific magical skill (tarot, herbalism, etc.)
- One book about magical ethics and philosophy
- One journal for your own magical experiences and insights

As you grow, add:

- Books about specific magical traditions that interest you
- Historical texts about magic and witchcraft
- Books by practitioners from diverse cultural backgrounds
- Advanced texts about specialized magical skills
- Books about integrating spirituality with activism and social justice

CREATING SACRED SPACE ON A BUDGET

Free or Low-Cost Sacred Space Ideas:

- Use a windowsill, dresser top, or corner of a room
- Repurpose household items as altar pieces
- Collect natural materials from walks outside
- Use drawings or printouts instead of expensive artwork

- Make your own tools from craft supplies
- Create digital altars if physical space is limited

Sacred Space for Closeted or Cautious Practitioners:

- Keep magical items in a decorative box or bag
- Use subtle symbols that others won't recognize
- Create portable altar setups that can be quickly assembled and put away
- Use phone apps for spell timing, moon phases, and other magical information
- Practice visualization and energy work that requires no physical tools

SEASONAL CELEBRATIONS AND HOLIDAYS

Traditional Pagan Holidays (adapt as desired):

- Samhain (October 31) - Honoring ancestors, releasing what no longer serves
- Winter Solstice (December 21) - Celebrating returning light, setting intentions
- Imbolc (February 2) - Preparing for spring, blessing creative projects
- Spring Equinox (March 21) - Balance, new growth, fresh starts
- Beltane (May 1) - Fertility, creativity, passionate connection
- Summer Solstice (June 21) - Peak energy, celebration, manifestation
- Lughnasadh (August 1) - First harvest, appreciating achievements
- Fall Equinox (September 23) - Second harvest, gratitude, preparation

LGBTQ+-Specific Observances:

- Pride Month (June) - Celebration, visibility, community
- Coming Out Day (October 11) - Courage, authenticity, support
- Transgender Day of Remembrance (November 20) - Memorial, solidarity, action
- Transgender Day of Visibility (March 31) - Celebration, awareness, advocacy
- Spirit Day (October) - Anti-bullying, youth support, purple solidarity

MAGICAL ETHICS AND SAFETY

Ethical Guidelines for LGBTQ+ Practitioners:

- Focus on your own growth rather than controlling others
- Respect consent in all magical workings
- Consider the potential impact of your magic on others
- Work for justice while avoiding harm when possible
- Honor the traditions you learn from without appropriating
- Share knowledge generously while respecting intellectual propert
- Support LGBTQ+ magical practitioners and communities

Safety Considerations:

- Never use magic as a substitute for medical care, legal protection, or practical action
- Be cautious about sharing your magical practice

with people who might discriminate
- Trust your intuition about people and situations
- Have practical safety plans in addition to magical protection
- Seek professional help for serious mental health or safety concerns
- Remember that being LGBTQ+ can make you vulnerable in some situations regardless of magical protection

CONTINUING EDUCATION AND GROWTH

Ways to Deepen Your Practice:

- Attend LGBTQ+-affirming Pagan gatherings and festivals
- Take online courses about specific magical skills
- Find a mentor who understands both magic and LGBTQ+ experience
- Join or start a local magical study group
- Attend workshops at metaphysical shops or community centers
- Practice divination systems like tarot or runes
- Learn about herbalism, astrology, or other magical specialties
- Study the history of magic and witchcraft in different cultures

Teaching and Mentoring Others:

- Share your knowledge with newer practitioners
- Write about your experiences for LGBTQ+ spiritual communities
- Offer to facilitate workshops or discussion groups
- Mentor young LGBTQ+ people interested in magical practice

- Create online content about queer magical practice
- Volunteer with LGBTQ+ organizations that welcome spiritual perspectives

ADAPTING PRACTICES FOR DIFFERENT LIVING SITUATIONS

For People Living with Non-Accepting Family:

- Focus on internal practices like visualization and meditation
- Use household items for magical purposes
- Practice in private spaces like bathrooms or bedrooms
- Keep magical materials hidden or disguised
- Use phone apps and online resources for guidance
- Connect with online communities for support

For People with Limited Mobility or Chronic Illness:

- Adapt physical practices for your energy and mobility levels
- Focus on visualization and intention rather than elaborate rituals
- Use voice-to-text for magical journaling if writing is difficult
- Create comfortable sacred spaces that accommodate your physical needs
- Practice self-compassion when you can't maintain consistent routines
- Connect with other disabled magical practitioners for support and ideas

For People in Temporary or Unstable Housing:

- Create portable magical kits that can travel with you

- Focus on practices that don't require permanent sacred space
- Use digital tools for magical timing and record-keeping
- Practice grounding and centering techniques that work anywhere
- Build relationships with magical community that can provide stability
- Adapt practices for whatever space you currently have available

BUILDING MAGICAL COMMUNITY

Starting a LGBTQ+ Magical Group:

- Begin with informal gatherings of interested friends
- Meet in homes, community centers, or LGBTQ+-friendly businesses
- Start with simple activities like full moon gatherings or seasonal celebrations
- Use social media to connect with potential members
- Partner with existing LGBTQ+ organizations for outreach
- Create inclusive ground rules that welcome practitioners at all levels

Online Community Building:

- Start social media groups focused on LGBTQ+ magical practice
- Host virtual gatherings for people who can't meet in person
- Create Discord servers or other platforms for ongoing discussion

- Organize online seasonal celebrations or magical workings
- Share resources and support for people building their practices
- Connect people in similar geographic areas who might want to meet offline

FINAL THOUGHTS: YOUR MAGICAL JOURNEY

This book is just the beginning of your magical journey. The practices, spells, and ideas here are meant to inspire and support you, but they're not the final word on what your magical practice should look like. Your queerness, your unique life experiences, and your personal spiritual insights are all valid contributions to the magical community.

As you grow in your practice, remember:

You belong in magical spaces. Your LGBTQ+ identity isn't something you need to hide or minimize to practice magic. It's an integral part of who you are and how you move through the world magically.

Your perspective matters. The magical community is enriched by diverse voices and experiences. Don't be afraid to share your insights, create new practices, or adapt existing ones to better serve LGBTQ+ folks.

Magic is both personal and political. Your practice of living authentically, loving boldly, and creating positive change in your own life contributes to a more magical world for everyone.

Growth is ongoing. You don't need to have everything figured out to begin practicing magic, and your practice will continue evolving throughout your life. Embrace the journey rather than rushing toward some imagined destination.

Community makes everything stronger. While magic

can be deeply personal, sharing the journey with others who understand your experiences makes the path richer and more sustainable.

Your magic matters. Whether you're just beginning to explore magical practice or you've been practicing for years, your unique approach to magic contributes something valuable to the world. Your spells, your rituals, your way of being magical—all of it matters.

The world needs more magic, and it especially needs the kind of transformative, authentic, justice-oriented magic that LGBTQ+ practitioners bring to spiritual communities. Your practice is both a gift to yourself and a gift to the world.

May your magic bring you joy, healing, growth, and authentic connection. May your practice support you in becoming ever more yourself. And may your authentic magical presence help create a world where all LGBTQ+ people can thrive.

Blessed be, and welcome to your magical life.

"Magic is not a practice. It is a living, breathing web of energy that, with our permission, can encase our every action."
- Dorothy Morrison

"The most magical thing you can be is yourself."
- Unknown

"We are the granddaughters of the witches you couldn't burn."
- Tish Thawer

"Your magic is not in your perfection. Your magic is in your willingness to grow."
- Rebecca Campbell

"The world needs your magic—your authentic, unapologetic, revolutionary magic." -
- Lisa Lister

www.ingramcontent.com/pod-product-compliance
Lightning Source LLC
Chambersburg PA
CBHW031157020426
42333CB00013B/702